Type Awesome

Jo Fox

www.typeawesome.co.uk

Copyright © Jo Fox 2020
All rights reserved

No part of this publication may be reproduced, distributed, or transmitted in any form or by any means, including photocopying, recording, or other electronic or mechanical methods, without the prior written permission of the publisher, except in the case of brief quotations embodied in reviews and certain other non commercial uses permitted by copyright law.
Independently Published.

ISBN: 9781838539061

Disclaimer

This book details the contributor's personal experiences with and opinions of Type 1 Diabetes, including their treatment and management of the condition. The author is not a healthcare provider or medical professional.

The author and publisher are providing this book and its contents on an "as is" basis and make no representations or warranties of any kind with respect to this book or its contents. The author and publisher disclaim all such representations and warranties. In addition, the author and publisher do not represent or warrant that the information accessible via this book is accurate, complete or current.

The statements made about products and services are purely the contributors own. They are not intended to diagnose, treat, cure, manage or prevent any medical condition or disease. Please consult with your own medical professional/s and/or healthcare providers before carrying out any suggestions and/or recommendations made in this book.

Except as specifically stated in this book, neither the author or publisher, nor any authors, contributors, or other representatives will be liable for damages arising out of or in connection with the use of this book.

This is a comprehensive limitation of liability that applies to all damages of any kind, including (without limitation) compensatory; direct, indirect or consequential damages; loss of data, income or profit; loss of or damage to property and claims of third parties.

You understand that this book is not intended as a substitute for medical advice. Consult your healthcare professionals before you begin any healthcare program, or change your lifestyle, diabetes treatment or management in anyway. Consult a professional to ensure that you are in good health and that the examples described in this book will not harm you.

This book provides content related to type 1 diabetes. As such, use of this book implies your acceptance of this disclaimer.

Contributors to this publication come from different countries; not all medications and products mentioned will be available in every territory.

Contents

Forward by Jo Fox	5
About Type 1 Diabetes	9
Chapter 1: Major Sir Frederick Grant Banting, M.C	14
Chapter 2: Jess Burton	36
Chapter 3: Glen Freeman	52
Chapter 4: Jade Byrne	64
Chapter 5: Jordan Thompson	73
Chapter 6: Lydia Parkhurst	84
Chapter 7 Laura Dunion	96
Chapter 8 - Mary Hayes	111
Chapter 9: Tilly-Rose Dade	123
Chapter 10: Rebecca Redmond	130
Chapter 11: About JDRF - a look at the latest research	141
Chapter 11: About The Pendsey Trust	152
Glossary	160

Forward by Jo Fox

My son was diagnosed in December, 2013, he was then aged just 6. I remember in hospital; the nurse came to give him an injection and I told her that he had just had one. She said she knew; this is how life is for us now, injections every few hours. The reality hit me, just like that. I came to learn that the injections are the easy bit, the hard bit is living with the anxiety Type 1 brings. The hard bit is comforting a 6-year-old who is crying because the book the hospital gave him says "Diabetes will not go away. You will have this for the rest of your life". The hard bit is knowing how to answer a 9-year-old when he asks if he is going to die in the night. The hard bit is the child been excluded from groups and clubs because of diabetes. The hard bit is the child coming home from school with 29 letters of apology from the class, who were excluding him and thinking that they can catch diabetes.

A Type 1 Diabetes diagnosis affects the whole family. It is incredibly isolating, especially at first. Type 1 challenges everything you thought you knew about diabetes, there is so much to learn and it can be overwhelming at first. If you get it wrong, it can be deadly, so that is not an option. Everyone involved in the child's care needs to become a mathematician, dietician, doctor, nurse and psychologist overnight. This means school staff require training, as well as after school club staff, childminders, family members who look after the child and anyone who looks after them. All this is made worse by the misunderstandings and misconceptions society has about diabetes.

Just 3 months into diagnosis, we suddenly had support as another boy in the class was diagnosed. Our family went through the anxiety together with this other family, who we will forever be grateful to. Not everyone has this support and diabetes is very isolating.

The first few years after diagnosis I was very depressed and very anxious. I did used to worry about his future and whether I would ever let him walk home from school alone for the fear of hypo. I wondered whether he would ever be able to drive, or would diabetes make that difficult as people with Type 1 are already given a restrictive licence. I wondered how he would cope on school trips, especially when I wasn't there to help. No one can look after my boy as well as I can. I wondered if we would ever travel abroad as a family again, we like our extended trips to off-the-beaten track places. I wondered how we could ever just wake up and take off camping in our campervan, with diabetes making spontaneity difficult. I wondered if his future jobs and careers would be affected. I worried about his future, it is often hard to see beyond the next few hours of this cruel condition, especially when you are testing every two hours throughout the night. I would be awake throughout the night, feeling like the only person testing their child throughout the night. I would be crying a river of tears at 3am, because that's the only time my son wouldn't see me getting upset.

I started to look online for re-assurance, I wanted to know that if we put the work in, life will turn out well for my son. I wanted to read about people who were doing great things and living a full life, despite living alongside this condition. But, I would only find horror stories. I remember one story on a main diabetes website where a teenage girl recalled her residential school trip to France, she went into DKA whilst in Paris, was hospitalised and her parents had to fly out. It was touch and go, but she was OK in the end, hence she was telling the tale. I already knew bad things like this could happen; I had gone online for reassurance that I did not get.

Determined not to let diabetes stop us, we found ways for life to carry on. We fit diabetes into our life and just got on with it. We had no other choice. We became involved in the wonderfully supportive Type 1 Diabetes community, we met many people with Type 1 who were a great source of support. We met adults or older children who were diagnosed at a young age, they were very inspiring to us and helped us see that life goes on. I found great comfort and re-assurance meeting these people who have not let diabetes get in their way. Many people were just as successful as their peers, if not more so and some were at the top of their game. This was very different to the stories I had found online, the horror stories I had read about seemingly weren't as popular as these websites made out – although the risk is of course very real.

I realised there is certainly a lack of positive Type 1 Diabetes stories and role models for young people out there and online. It is time people with Type 1 diabetes were celebrated; someone needs to tell their tale and bring them into the spotlight, which is one of the purposes of this book – to celebrate the Type Awesome's who are battling this condition but still living a full life. Many people do not see the struggles they go through in order to carry on, the hurdles they have to overcome on a daily basis and it is time for that to change. Type Awesome is a collaboration of positive stories from awesome people who have to jump over these hurdles; celebrating their determination, resilience and indomitable spirit.

My son did start walking home from school with his friends; when he was old enough to do so, of course. He has friends and socialises out of school, thankfully so far the bullying was a one off incident. He is awesome at playing guitar and is musically gifted. He plays football, is especially good in goals and is a big fan of Leeds United. We still go on spontaneous trips in the campervan. We still travel abroad. We travelled thousands of miles around India, for a month, in 40c heat and entirely by train! He spoke in front of hundreds at a diabetes conference in India, inspiring other children with diabetes. In India, we had no major diabetes problems, but the year after we left ALL the diabetes supplies on a bus in Italy! We had a few hours worth of supplies with us, the rest was on a coach to Venice whilst we were in Lake Garda! It was our first day on a 10-day trip. But we got through it! We were 5 years in at this stage, so definitely not a rookie mistake, but mistakes happen and there is always a solution. My son went on activity, adrenaline fuelled residential school trips at ages 10 and 12, he had extremely good blood sugars the whole time he was there and did all the work himself with staff providing only moral support. I would say diabetes has not stopped us doing anything, it certainly makes some things more difficult and it gives us a lot to think about and plan for, but we don't let it stop us.

The other purpose of this book is to re-assure others, to show positive and real-life examples of people who have had amazing achievements despite fighting this relentless battle daily. A battle that is often hidden, or fought behind curtains or on the side-lines; a condition that is often misunderstood or misinterpreted. I hope by reading this book, parents of children with Type 1 will have some of their anxieties eased; that they will be inspired by these awesome people, it can be motivating to see how these people have overcome the challenges diabetes brings and achieved their dreams. Maybe young people too will feel motivated and inspired, these stories can help them if they feel diabetes is getting them down. For everybody else, I hope you learn more about this condition and how it impacts daily life. This is the book I wish someone had handed me seven years ago.

A book containing inspirational and motivational Type 1 diabetes stories. This is the book I wish I had been handed at diagnosis.

About Type 1 Diabetes

When we eat, the energy from the food goes into our bloodstream. Insulin is a hormone made by the pancreas, insulin's main function is to move the energy in the bloodstream around the body into the other essential organs. The role of insulin can be compared to a key that unlocks to move energy on from the blood to other body parts.

Everyone is insulin dependent; without it we will go into coma and death soon follows. Type 1 Diabetes happens when the immune system wrongly attacks the insulin producing beta cells in the pancreas. The body has no other way of making insulin, meaning energy from food remains locked in the blood stream. This causes blood sugars to elevate and symptoms of Type 1 Diabetes will at this stage be very noticeable. This means that when someone is diagnosed with Type 1 Diabetes, they have to inject insulin from that day on and for the rest of their life, as there is currently is no cure.

Blood sugar should be between 4 - 7 mmol, when it is above 14 the body is suffering and looks for other ways to find energy. One way the body gets energy is by burning its own fat, this process produces a chemical called ketone and a build up ketones leads to a condition called Keto Acidosis (DKA), which is a diabetic coma. Coma leads to death. The body can start this process within hours of having high blood sugars. Insulin needs to be given to prevent this. It is not unusual to have blood sugars in the 20's or even 30s, even people with excellent control can experience this sometimes and could be for no apparent reason. Insulin is the only way to bring blood sugar down to avoid **DKA**. In the longer term, high blood sugars can cause heart and kidney problems, serious eyesight issues and painful foot problems and this can lead to limb amputations, blindness and heart & kidney failure.

People with Type 1 Diabetes must test their blood and inject themselves with insulin multiple times a day in order to stay alive. Every single thing they eat or drink has to be weighed, measured and carb counted, then insulin is matched to the number of carbs. Many other factors affect blood sugars too, including hormones, puberty, menstruation, growth spurts, other illnesses, viruses, infections, other medications, anxiety, excitement, depression, stress, adrenaline, sleep, routine (or disruption to routine), the temperature, the weather and even the day of the week!

The human body needs sugar to function properly. When the blood sugar drops below 4, this is considered hypoglycaemic (hypo) and is a true medical emergency for a person with diabetes. A hypo can easily happen to anyone with type 1 diabetes, even those with good control can have several hypo's a week. Hypo's happen when blood sugar has accidently dropped too low and the immediate treatment is sugar. Symptoms of hypo can include; shaking, fatigue, sweating, hunger, behaviour changes, confusion, anger, dizziness, tingling, anxiousness, palpitation's and looking pale. If not treated, the person can have seizures and become unconscious. A person who is hypoglycaemic may not be cognitively aware, this is because they do not have enough sugar in their body for the brain to function properly. A person with diabetes should always carry sugary snacks with them; such as glucose or dextrose tablets, sugary sweets, Lucozade or full sugar soda. Once enough sugar is consumed and it will then raise their blood sugar to a safe level.

Hypoglycaemia can happen for a lot of reasons; meals could be delayed or missed, the carb content of the meal might be different to that calculated, the person might have not quite eaten everything on their plate, but also things like exercise, extreme heat or cold, adrenaline rush or stomach bugs can cause hypo's.

It is impossible for a person with Type 1 Diabetes to have the correct amount of insulin all the time, so it is inevitable that hypo's and hyper's (high blood sugars) are going to occur on a regular basis. The job of the person with diabetes (or their carers) is to try and keep blood sugars within safe levels by trying to manage the highs and lows. Insulin doses must be monitored and reviewed on a regular basis. No two days are the same; if Johnny has a banana on Monday he might need 4 units of insulin, if Johnny has the same sized banana on Wednesday he might need 8 units, the same banana on Friday and he might be OK to eat the banana without any insulin at all.

Type 1 Diabetes facts and Fiction

- Type 1 is NOT diet or lifestyle related.
- Anyone can get Type 1, but it often develops in childhood.
- Insulin is NOT a cure.
- A person cannot reverse Type 1
- A child will not "grow out of it", unfortunately!
- Type 1 requires constant monitoring, even through the night!
- It is a 24/7 condition, never gives a day off, even at Christmas.
- A person with Type 1 must test their bloods and inject insulin MANY times a day in order to stay alive, or use a CGM and pump.
- That is the easy bit, the hard bit is knowing how much to inject, slightly too much or too little can be very dangerous.
- People with Type 1 can eat anything at all that they want to. They can even eat cake, chocolate and sweets.
- Type 1 does not require the person to follow any special diet and no foods are eliminated, in fact, some carbs can stabilise blood sugar and at other times, sugary foods can save their life.
- A person with Type 1 can eat ANYTHING, even cake!
- Type 1 is a very tough condition to live with.
- Type 1 affects the whole family.
- An insulin pump is NOT a cure - the wearer has to give the pump all its commands throughout the day.
- A pump can actually take more monitoring than injections and can be more dangerous if something goes wrong.
- Type 1's might need a rest sometimes, but they are not using their condition as an excuse. This is a tiring condition.
- Type 1 should not be used to make fun of someone, nor is it a source of jokes.
- Type 1 affects every aspect of the person's life.
- Type 1 never stabilises, or settles down.

- Type 1 makes any common illness much worse, stomach bugs especially can be deadly.
- 40% of people with T1 diabetes also have an eating disorder.
- Many also have depression, anxiety or other mental health diagnoses .
- Diabetes burn out is a real condition, it is tiring constantly managing this condition.
- Type 1's have to carry life saving equipment with them ALL THE TIME.
- Type 1's don't want to hear about your next door neighbours grandsons next door neighbours cat who also has diabetes.
- Or that your great Uncle had his leg off because of diabetes.
- Type 1 is never like Type 2 (even if the person with T2 injects!)
- Type 1 can not be cured; not even with cinnamon, herbs or the "plant of Africa."
- Insulin is the only potentially fatal drug where the user calculates the dosage, even if the user is a child.
- Knowing how much insulin to give is an educated guess!
- There is an incredibly supportive Type 1 Community
- **People with Type 1 Diabetes are Awesome and Superhuman!**

Chapter 1

"Consider it my gift to mankind"

Sir Frederick Banting, by Jo Fox

Before meeting the awesome people in this book who have achieved amazing things, despite their battles with diabetes, lets meet the amazing man who made their lives possible, Sir Frederick Banting.

Banting was born on 14th November, 1891, on a farm in Alliston, Ontario, which is approximately 40 miles north of Toronto, Canada. Banting had a happy childhood on the farm; the youngest of his 3 brothers and 1 sister, so he always had other children to play with, but he was shy as a child. The Banting family was religious. Fred's parents, Margaret Grant and William Banting, were hardworking people and of the Methodist persuasion.

Banting was a hardworking and conscientious student. Although he did not excel and had to work hard to get average grades, he always gave his best effort to anything he put his mind to. It is thought that he first had the idea to become a Doctor during his childhood. He famously recalls a time on his way home from school when he saw two men fall from great height off some scaffolding. The men were on the ground; one was still and quiet, whilst the other initially moved his arms and then lay there still. Banting went to fetch the local doctor, who came to the scene just a few minutes later. The doctor tended to the men and skilfully attended to their broken limbs, cuts and bleeding, but mainly, everyone was relieved at the presence of the doctor and in awe of his ability to help. From that day on, Banting decided he would one day become a doctor and used to say that giving service in the medical field is the greatest way to give service in life.

Frederick Banting also had a passion for the liberal arts, especially painting. In 1910, he enrolled in a general arts programme at Victoria College at The University of Toronto, where he became a member of the Vic Glee Club. He had a powerful baritone voice and would participate in concerts at the University. Despite Fred's (as he then preferred to be known) passion and ability at art, he failed his first year of college, and although he re-enrolled to repeat the year, he had already made the decision to become a doctor. Leaving the arts wasn't a decision to be taken lightly; Banting's parents had hoped he would join the ministry, but the Methodist minister, Reverend Peter Addison, told Banting to follow his own path and do what his heart was telling him was the right thing. Banting chose medicine and, with the blessing of his parents, he enrolled in medical school in September of 1913.

Banting was an average student in medical school. Although he worked very hard, sometimes he would barely scrape a pass, but in other areas of his studies he would excel and pass with flying colours. At best, Banting was considered to be an average medical student overall. At this point, he was more interested in gaining surgical experience than in scientific research, and he also spent a lot of time playing rugby with the university team.

Banting the War Hero

War had been brewing in Europe and finally broke out in 1914. Campus life changed somewhat. Fred applied to the Canadian military but was held back from joining due to his poor eyesight. There was another way Fred could help on the western front, by becoming a military medic as there was a great shortage of them. Banting's intake at the University of Toronto could chose to be fast tracked through medical school, effectively condensing their final year of study into the summer break. This option was provided for those who wished to help the war effort by serving in the medical corps. Banting graduated medical school on 4th December, 1916, and enlisted as a Medical Field Officer in the Canadian Army Medical Corps on 5th December, 1916. Medics were in high demand in the battlefields of Europe. Banting's role was to tend to the injured. He travelled to France with the Canadian 13th Field Regiment. At first, Banting served as a relief medical officer working in casualty clearing stations, dressing stations, and receiving in wounded officers who required medical care. Hungry for some action himself, he transferred to the 44th division, 4th Canadian Corps, where he was moved to the centre of the fighting in the town of Arras.

One of Banting's jobs was to perform surgery on a soldier who had a throat abscess which needed cutting open and draining. Banting had to perform this procedure as an emergency, and he was so concerned for the life of the injured soldier that he personally kept a bedside vigil to ensure there was no haemorrhage. Thankfully, there were no complications of any kind, and the soldier made a full recovery, returning just 48 hours later to the battlefield.

It was 27th September, 1918, the Battle of Canal du Nord, when allied troops came under enemy attack. Heavy shell fire came over, resulting in many men being wounded or killed. Banting himself was badly wounded. Shrapnel from an exploding shell ripped through his right arm causing a severe injury. Despite this, Banting continued to treat injured soldiers and tend to their wounds, which was against the advice of his seniors who were pleading with him to stop. After 17 hours of dressing the wounds of other soldiers whilst injured himself, Banting gave in so that he could finally receive care for his own wound. Banting was sent to the Canadian Red Cross Special Hospital in Buxton, England, where he remained for three months. During this time, Banting almost had to have his arm amputated, which shows how severe his own wounds were, yet he selflessly considered other soldiers' needs to be more important than his own. Banting left hospital several months later and returned home to Toronto, as by then the war had ended. Upon his return to Canada, Banting received the Military Cross, the second highest order, for his heroism whilst under fire.

Post War Years

Banting found it exhilarating to know that he had skills needed to save lives. He felt he had proved his worth as a man and a doctor, after initially thinking his medical training was deficient due to rushing through the final year. After official discharge from the Army in the summer of 1919, Banting went to work at the Toronto Hospital for Sick Children. At this stage, Banting was still only a junior doctor and needed to gain surgical experience. He undertook routine operations on children such as appendectomies, tonsillectomies and fracture repairs. Banting became a talented and skilful surgeon and was very popular with his patients, but he could not remain at the children's' hospital as it had only been a temporary placement for him to fully qualify and gain experience as a surgeon. With no job openings at the hospital he left and moved to London, Ontario, where he opened a general medical practice.

London was a new place to Banting. He didn't have connections there and he wasn't known as a widely experienced doctor, so his income suffered. Banting slowly built up some income from tending to his patients, but as it was summer and people generally needed doctors in the cold Canadian winters, Banting needed to look for another source of income. Banting undertook a role lecturing in physiology and human anatomy at the University of Western Ontario. Working at the University also allowed Banting access to the medical library, where he would read medical journals and advance his knowledge.

Insulin and diabetes

In autumn of 1920, Professor Miller, of Western University, asked Banting to prepare a lecture for his students on metabolism and carbohydrates. Not knowing too much about the subject himself, as he claimed to have never worked with patients with diabetes, he had to read up on the subject himself. Banting went to the university library and read all the journals and textbooks he could find about the role of the pancreas and diabetes. Banting learned that the insulin producing cells were known as the 'islets of Langerhans', and when there is a problem with these, the patients die. Functioning islet cells prevented diabetes.

Banting went home and considered what he had learned: a secretion from the islet cells is needed in order for the body to metabolise carbohydrates. Without carbohydrates we die from malnutrition. People with Type 1 Diabetes appear to be missing this substance that is released by the islet cells, so the sugar from carbohydrate cannot be metabolised and the patient dies from "sugar disease". In bed that night, Banting could not sleep and kept thinking about the article. In the early hours of the morning, he had an idea which he believed was a solution to the problem of diabetes. Banting could not get the idea from his head and for fear he would have forgotten it the next morning, he wrote it down. The 25 words he wrote down led to a leap in treatment for diabetes.

"Diabetus ligate pancreatic ducts of dogs keep dogs alive until acini degenerates leaving islets. Try to isolate internals secretion of these to relieve glycosuria."

Frederick Banting, 1920

Banting basically had the idea to isolate pancreatic cells, collect the secretion, and then inject it into patients with Type 1 to lower their blood sugar. Banting went to Professor Mellor with his idea and asked if he could research it at Western University, but they did not have the resources to accommodate such extensive research and had no facilities for animal experimentation on that level. Professor Mellor helped Banting to develop his idea, though, by referring him to JJ R McLeod at the University of Toronto. McLeod was an expert in the field of carbohydrate metabolism.

McLeod initially thought it was a bad idea and he had many concerns. Banting was still a young and inexperienced doctor with very limited scientific research and what's more, he knew very little about diabetes, the pancreas and carbohydrate metabolism. Banting was enthusiastic and persistent, and eventually McLeod allowed him to use his facilities to conduct some initial research. McLeod lent the research project a laboratory, equipment, and animals upon which to experiment. He provided Banting with two further people who could help him develop his idea, Charles Best, a student assistant, and J. B. Collip, a bio-chemist from the University of Alberta, who had been on placement in Toronto.

Banting would perform pancreatectomies on dogs, whilst Best would use his skills to test the dogs' urine as sugar levels started rising in the dogs. Banting would perform many experiments on the pancreases he removed and would try to isolate the secretion that was believed to be essential to metabolise carbohydrates. McLeod's role was monitoring and advising on carbohydrates and anatomy. Collip's job was to advise on bio-chemistry. Further into the studies, Banting would not remove the pancreas, but ligate it instead to allow the secretion to collect.

In July, 1921, a dog pancreas was dissected and the secretion extracted. Five mL of this secretion was removed and injected into a dog with no pancreas. The dog's blood sugar improved, but the effects did not last long and the dog died the next morning. The results, however, were very significant, and they provided evidence that the secretion had been correctly identified and isolated. Banting called the secretion an "anti-diabetic solution" and later "isletin" – named after the islet cells in the pancreas.

Experiments continued by Banting and Best, highly monitoring dogs and constantly testing the levels of sugar in their bodies by testing their urine sugar levels. Another dog with no pancreas was given repeated injections throughout the day in order to keep the sugar levels down, and the dog remained healthy and free of symptoms of diabetes. The dog, Marjorie, lived for 70 days and was injected with isletin every few hours.

McLeod was impressed with the progress the team had made, but tensions were often strained in the lab. Banting could get angry and would accuse Best of not taking accurate urine tests. Best sometimes stormed out. Both Banting and Best had devoted all their time to the research, with Banting giving up his clinic in London, whilst McLeod did not want other ongoing projects at the university to suffer. Banting was struggling financially, with no reliable source of income and he had to sell his car to fund his living expenses. Banting and Best started demanding salaries, more dogs for experiments, and lab assistants. Tensions were high and it was believed Banting was suffering from Post-Traumatic Stress Disorder (PTSD), possibly a result of his heroic actions in the war. McLeod was very reluctant to give in to Banting's requests, but eventually offered him everything he was demanding. One of the conditions was that he changed the name of isletin to insulin, which was considered a much easier word to pronounce.

In October of 1921, Banting and Best continued their work on dogs, but realized that in order to be successful they would need a constant supply of insulin and dogs would simply not provide enough to meet the demand. Cattle were brought in, pancreases removed, and insulin could be isolated on a much bigger scale due to their size.
The insulin solution was injected into several dogs. Bovine insulin was keeping the dogs alive, but before the solution could be tested on humans it needed to be purified. Collip was responsible for this process, and in December, 1921, he began work to do this, and experiments with purified insulin extracts were successfully repeated on rabbits. The solution was now ready to be tested on humans.

Banting had long been dreaming of playing a key role in testing his insulin solution on people who were suffering from diabetes. Patients with diabetes were required; Toronto Hospital for Sick Children had a ward full of 52 patients who were in, or close to, diabetic coma, their parents keeping vigil at their bedside waiting for the inevitable to happen. In the afternoon of 11th January, 1922, Leonard Thompson received the first insulin injection; no benefits were observed and Leonard developed an abscess at the injection site. The extract was not pure enough.

The team went back to the lab disheartened, yet determined to make their experiment successful in treating patients with diabetes. Tensions were again high, and Banting believed McLeod, who was the more experienced doctor and researcher, wanted to steal the idea from him and claim all the credit for the work. After some arguments in the lab, the co-researchers agreed to work together, and a kind of peace treaty was agreed allowing them to collaborate and purify the insulin that had failed on 11th January.

Just 12 days later, on 23rd January, 1920, Leonard Thompson was injected a second time with Collip's purified insulin. This time, there was immediate improvement in blood sugar levels and further patients were injected with no apparent side effects. Other patients on the ward were treated, and as the last were injected the first were miraculously awakening from their diabetic comas. To this day, this is still known and referred to as medicine's modern miracle. What an event this must have been to witness and how pleased must Banting have been to witness the miraculous outcome of his discovery. Leonard Thompson's health improved and he went on to live for 13 more years, dying of pneumonia at age 26.

Banting at this time was still in debt and not earning enough money to get by comfortably. He was suffering from depression, anger outbursts and anxiety and was still plagued by nightmares from the horrific events and scenes he witnessed in the war. Toronto General Hospital offered him a job working as a doctor on a ward with 32 patients with diabetes. This not only helped him solve his financial problems but also provided him with the opportunity to continue his work and research into diabetes.

Banting became famous overnight; his colleagues in the worldwide medical and scientific institutions sent their praises and congratulations.
Banting's photo appeared on the front covers of newspapers, magazines and journals worldwide. Many scientific and medical organisations made him an honorary member, he received many awards, prizes, medals and honorary titles all over the world.

Banting would be stopped whenever he went out, people with diabetes and their families would simply want to thank him for his work and for saving their lives. Invitations were plentiful, with offers to give talks, speeches and lectures about his work. In England, he was received by the monarch, King George V, and he was made a Knight Commander of the Order of the British Empire (KBE) in 1934 for his services to medicine. In America he appeared on the front cover of Time magazine. Banting, however, did not enjoy the fame and did not like a fuss. He was a very modest man and did not want to be remembered for his titles and awards, but for his research in the medical field. Banting just wanted to get on with his life and work; he had many other interests to pursue both in the medical field and in his personal life.

In October of 1923, Banting and McLeod were awarded the Nobel Prize in Physiology and Medicine. Banting was granted the credit for the discovery and McLeod for being constant throughout the experiments. The four co-researchers shared out the Nobel Prize money equally, although Banting and Best donated theirs to diabetic research projects at the University of Toronto, in order to further develop understanding of the condition. As of writing (October, 2020) Banting still remains the youngest person ever to receive the Nobel Prize for Physiology and Medicine, as he was just 32 years old when the prize was awarded to him.

On October 9th, 1923, Banting, Best & Collip were granted the patent for insulin, or technically the "*extract obtainable from mammalian pancreas or from the related glans in fishes, useful in the treatment of diabetes mellitus and a method of preparing it*". U.S Patent no 1,469,994 was granted to the three co-discoverers, which meant they now owned the sole rights to produce insulin. It is worth noting that Banting was not a rich man at this point; he had lived in relative poverty and even had to sell his car whilst conducting the experiments in order to make ends meet. Banting was not a well-known doctor or researcher, so his experiments did not attract the usual grants or subsidies that those of senior medics would. A substantial amount of money could be made from selling the patent to a drug company, but Banting did not want insulin to be unaffordable. He wanted to make sure it was accessible to everyone who needed it. If drug companies owned the patent, only the wealthy would be able to afford it, which would leave the poorer people in society without access to it. For this reason, Banting and Best decided to give the patent away to the University of Toronto, who made a token payment of $1 for it. Banting had been offered millions of dollars for the patent from multi-national pharmaceutical corporations, but he turned them down, claiming insulin was his "gift to mankind." Toronto's gift to the world was also insulin and to this present day, the city is home to significant research surrounding diabetes.

Banting as an artist

Banting struggled to cope with the pressures of his new-found fame, in 1932 he divorced his first wife, Marion Robertson, after a 6 year marriage in which they had a son, William. Divorce was still considered a sin in Canada at this time. Banting's fame resulted in further media exposure which he did not like; he claimed the media were more interested in writing about his divorce than they were writing about his medical discoveries, or his art work, which was another field in which he expelled, despite having failed art college. Banting was still struggling with mental health issues as a result of his experiences in The Great War.

Painting was Banting's escape from the world, it was his refuge from the professional world which was starting to put pressure on him to make another ground-breaking discovery. Painting was a creative outlet in which Banting felt he could express himself, release stress and possibly he used art as a form of therapy to help him deal with Post Traumatic Stress Disorder. Banting was an incredibly talented landscape artist and found solace in creativity. Painting landscapes first became important to Banting during his time living in London, Ontario, when he had set up his clinic but didn't have many patients. Never one to be idle, as a way to occupy his time, Banting began to paint, draw and carve wood in order to pass the time.

Banting visited an art store on Dundas Street, which was close to his clinic and he loved a boating print they had on display called The Landing. Banting practiced his drawing skills by copying The Landing, along with several other pictures he saw in various art books. A laundry store nearby would save the inlay card from the shirt packets for him to draw on, this saved Banting money on buying his own paper supplies. Local artists congregated at the art store and one lady, Mary Healey, a talented portrait artist, encouraged Banting to try painting with oils. From that moment on, Banting discovered his calling as an artist and became a very talented landscape oil painter.

Banting joined Toronto's Arts and Letters Club in 1925, he found camaraderie and friendship in the Group of Seven landscape painters. The Group of Seven were a group of renowned Canadian landscape artists whose work was very popular in the 1920's. Banting became good friends with one of the seven, A. Y. Jackson, with whom he shared a love of Canadian art and similar experiences of fighting in World War One. Banting and Jackson were lifelong friends and would take regular trips together around the vast terrain of Canada; painting landscapes out west in the Rockies, arctic icebergs in the Inuit communities to the north, the snowbound Quebec villages or Great Slave Lake in the Northwest Territories. It would often be so cold that their paint and brushes froze over!

Banting enjoyed the freedom of painting Canada's vast wilderness, he cherished the brotherhood he shared with A.Y. Jackson. In 1927, the artistic pair were invited to accompany the crew of the government steamship *S.S. Beothic,* on a two month arctic supply expedition. The two embraced the opportunity and created some fine art work on that trip, with Jackson acting as a mentor to Banting, who could often get frustrated with his perceived lack of progress. Banting committed to improving his technique on that trip and apparently, whenever he had finished a piece of work, he would take it to Jackson and ask "Now, what is wrong with it?"

Banting matured as an artist and he could see similarities between his art and his work; both science and art involved experimenting with techniques, either in a lab looking for scientific truths, or in the art world by experimenting with techniques in order to capture the world and create art. Jackson suggested jokingly that Banting should swap his microscope for paintbrushes, to which Banting responded that once he reached his 50th birthday he would happily turn to art full time and leave scientific discoveries to the younger generation. Banting left the following entry in his diary in 1930, *"it is a great country. The more I think of the city, the more I want to live in the country, and the more I think of being a professor of research, the more I want to be an artist or something else with more work and less responsibility"*

In the 1930's, Banting had his work displayed in various exhibitions at Toronto's Hart House Gallery and was by then a very well-known amateur artist. A humble man, just as he was in his scientific work, Banting often gave away the paintings and sometimes used the alias "Frederick Grant" in order to avoid publicity. Painting was Banting's escape from a world where he felt pressure and struggled to handle the fame his insulin discovery had brought him. Painting gave him a creative outlet, some peace of mind and was therapeutic, but he had no intention to become a famous artist.

Banting's last sketching trip was in 1938 when he went to St. Tite des Caps, Quebec, his work was so good that it was mistaken for Jackson's, even by art critics! Sadly, Banting never realized his dream of retiring at 50 to become a full-time artist as his life was tragically ended at age 49, as we will read later in this chapter.

Other Research Work

The Department of Medical Research at the University of Toronto were constructing a new building opposite the hospital which would be home to new state of the art scientific research laboratories. The University needed a name for the new department and wanted to honour Banting by calling it the Banting Institute. Of course, been the humble man he was, Banting did not agree to this and objected outright, but eventually the University went ahead anyway as they wanted to showcase Banting to the world, doing so would attract research grants for the new department. The Banting Institute was opened in 1930, Fred Banting took the whole of the top floor of the building for his research space. By this time, he had also been given an annual payment for life by the Canadian Government, who gave him permission to carry out any research he desired in any medical field.

Silicosis is a lung disease that occurs after inhaling particles of silica mineral dust, the condition was prevalent in miners across Canada at the time. Banting and Professor Haultain, a professor of Engineering, set out together to discover the relationship between mining and medicine. Banting had many questions; why does rock dust cause nodular fibrosis in miners? Which minerals are responsible? What is the relationship between rock dust and the lung, which is constantly moving during the mining process? Do horses, used in mines have silicosis? Can silicosis be treated or prevented?

Banting and Haultain conducted research into the effects of different chemical compounds on the silica, but they had mixed results. Banting found that alkaline partially dissolved the silica particles and hypothesised that an alkaline solution might help the body rid of silica via the kidneys. At the time, chemical methods were not sensitive enough to provide Banting with valid results, but his work led to other researchers within the department eventually continuing his work in silicosis. Banting had instigated this work and is still credited with discovering what is thought as the biggest breakthrough in silicosis knowledge and treatment.

In 1933, the Banting & Best Institute, the mining industry and Department of Industrial Hygiene worked together under Bantings suggestion to share knowledge and collaborate on research. It was discovered that the presence of certain gases in the mine air could accelerate silicosis. The work Banting supervised in his laboratory discovered how the lungs of miners retained and eliminated dust, which meant improvements could be made as to how the dust was identified and measured. New knowledge was gained from studying tissue reaction made by minerals from dust found in the mines.

By 1936, it was clearly understood which minerals were present in which Ontario mines, the silica dust alone could be responsible for fibrosis of the lung. Silicosis could be prevented by stopping the dust from entering the lungs, or by preventing silica acid forming. Banting was then part of a team who discovered that aluminium dust could be used as an anti-dote to silica; if the miners inhaled aluminium dust they could prevent and/or treat silicosis. Banting was a great leader throughout the silicosis research, he worked well with others and enjoyed co-ordinating teams of researchers. Banting visited the mines and enjoyed meeting the miners, on one occasion at Hollinger Mine, he was presented with a large quartz containing gold. He did not think he was worthy of keeping the entire sample, so he had it cut in half and donated the other half to the Royal Ontario Museum.

Another research interest of Banting's was heart failure, he conducted studies on the impact of injecting acetylcholine into animals with cardiac failure. It was found that acetylcholine could constrict blood vessels in animals. But Banting's main area of research interest at this time was cancer and he wanted to start oncological research. Banting wanted to find a cure for cancer, or at least a treatment that would save the lives of cancer patients in the same way insulin had done for patients with diabetes.

Working with colleague in England, William G. Eye, Banting discovered that a sarcoma can be caused by certain viruses, but then could be transmitted to others by injecting cells from one animal to another formerly cancer free animal. Banting was fascinated with this and knew that he could create cancer in animals in his lab, then he could reverse the process and look at ways into stop the cancer developing; maybe with a vaccine, secretion or antibody. On this occasion, the experiments were not successful, but Banting was not put off from further experiments into cancer and is credited with advancing knowledge in the treatment of sarcoma, although some of the work he supervised and led teams.

As the first Canadian Nobel Laureate, Banting was expected to travel internationally to conferences and give updates on his research. He spent a lot of time in the 1930's travelling and he was especially proud of his trip to the U.S.S.R, where he met the famous Physiologist Ivan Pavlov, who had an experimental research lab. Pavlov told Banting about Russia's social medicine programme, which worked like a National Health Service, the Canadian was highly impressed with the idea of a free at point of use health service and this gives some insight into his political views.

World War Two

In 1937, Banting married Henrietta Ball, his second wife, but this was also the year in which he became interested in biological warfare and how the enemy could spread disease. When World War Two broke in 1939, Banting conducted medical research into aviation medicine; studying the effects of velocity, high speeds, rapid descents and aerial manoeuvres used in combat and how these affected the human body. Banting's work in aviation medicine contributed to the development of the G-Suit, also known as an Anti-Gravity or Anti-G Suit. An Anti-G Suit is a flight suit worn by aviators who are subjected to high levels of acceleration force, this causes blood to pool in the lower part of the body during acceleration and as a result, the brain is deprived of oxygen and the pilot passes out. There had been many fatal accidents caused by the pilot blacking out after manoeuvres involving acceleration force. As war was raging, G-Suits were then put into use to prevent pilots of bomber planes from passing out.

G-Suits later made space exploration possible as astronauts are subjected to the same effects as pilots, but the G-Suit was adapted for space exploration as further forces are also present. Aircraft pilots for NATO have used G-Suits since the 1950's and still do today. Banting contributed towards the development of the suit, the initial prototype he was involved in bringing to market is still used today, for both aeronautical and space use. Again, the legacy of this amazing man's work extends for generations beyond his own lifetime and is still saving many lives nearly 100 years later.

War was still raging in Europe, Banting insisted in serving in the second world war, just as he had done in the first. The Canadian Government would not permit him to go to the front lines again as he was not only considered a national treasure, but his work on biological and aviation medicine used in warfare was also important for the war effort. It was also thought that in his late forties, Banting might not be fit enough for the front line.

During World War Two, he was promoted to the rank of Major, which made his official title Major Sir Frederick Banting, M.C, and he worked in an advisory role for the National Research Council of Canada (NRC). Banting's main role during the second world war was to work with the British and Canadian medical teams to ensure good working relationships were created and maintained. Banting concentrated on biological and chemical warfare, the focus of his research was to find better treatments for injuries such as mustard gas burns. To fully experience the medical condition and the treatment he had developed, Banting gave himself a mustard gas burn on his leg!

Major Banting believed that Britain was not paying enough attention to the threat of biological warfare from the enemy. He used his influence and reputation to create awareness of the risks to the British Government, the result was the setting up of a Micro-Biological Research Centre in the UK.

Death

On February 20th, 1941, Banting and two colleagues boarded a Hudson Bomber, Flight T-9449, to travel to the U.K, where he was to advise the British Government on chemical warfare, whilst there, he was to pick up sensitive research records and bring them back to Canada.

Sadly, not long after take-off, the plane experienced a malfunctioning oil cooler which caused the starboard engine to fail. The Pilot, Captain MacKey, made attempts to return to Gander airport, Newfoundland, where the flight had taken off just minutes before, these attempts were futile as the second engine also failed.
Knowing that the plane was about to crash, McKey suggested Banting and colleagues jump to try save themselves, but the didn't. It could be that Banting was now 49 years old and jumping out of a plane did not seem attractive. Or maybe he did not want to jump in the dark, not being able to see where the trees were or even of how
high up they were. Captain MacKey then attempted to land the plane on the frozen Seven Mile Pond, Newfoundland, but the aircraft was now out of control and clipped the trees. Unfortunately, the bomber came crashing down just meters away from a potentially
 safe landing place. The he crew died on impact but Banting survived along with Captain MacKey. The Captain walked to try
and find help, Banting was still conscious at this time, although he

27

did have a serious head injury.

Newfoundland is a very remote area of the world, but the community of Musgrave Harbour is approximately 10 miles from the crash site. A group of four hunters were taking a week-long rabbit hunting trip when their attention was drawn to a plane circling the sky. The plane was a search and rescue aircraft which had dropped paper notes from the air, the notes stated that a plane had crashed just one mile away and assistance was required as at least one man had survived and required help. The pilot of the aircraft then dropped another note which asked the men to follow underneath the path of the plane in order to reach the crash site. Upon finding the location of this tragic accident, the four men came across Captain Joseph Mackey, who was eating chocolate and wrapped up in a sleeping bag and sitting against a rock. The sleeping bag and chocolate bars had been dropped by the rescue plane earlier in the day. Captain Mackay would require medical attention and was eventually transferred from the crash site to the town of Musgrave Harbour by sledge, a journey of 10 miles!

The search and rescue plane had also dropped paper notes throughout the town of Musgrave Harbour, so residents there were aware of the crash and the location where help was required. Search and rescue parties were sent out to Seven Mile Pond, the bodies of the two crew were recovered immediately, but Banting's body could not be found. Three days after the accident, Banting's body was discovered preserved in the deep snow a mile away from the accident site. It is thought that his delirious state of mind and serious head injury had caused him to wander away. Banting's official cause of death was hypothermia, caused by exposure to the extreme cold, but the head injury might have also been a major contributing factor. It is thought that Banting had survived for up to 24 hours after the crash.

Captain Mackey was taken to a private home in Musgrave Harbour, where a resident who was a nurse set up an emergency clinic and provided medical care and attention to MacKey the best she could. After 3 days, Mackey was well enough to be airlifted to the larger town of Gander 30 miles away, which had a hospital that could provide the specialist care and rehabilitation he required. Captain Mackey eventually made a full recovery. MacKey later stated that it is a testament to Banting's character that the last thing he did was to help bandage the wounds MacKey had received in the accident, even though he was suffering himself.

The bodies of the men who perished in the accident were laid to rest in the Orange Lodge, Musgrave Harbour, until plans were made to return the men to their final resting place. It was at this point that the shocking news broke on the radio that one of the bodies recovered was the famous scientist, Sir Frederick Banting; the discoverer of insulin, Nobel Prize laureate, veteran of two world wars, recipient of the Military Cross (Canada's second highest accomplishment) for selfless and heroic work in the first world war and a Knight of the Order of the British Empire. Sir Frederick Banting, Canada's hero, a truly astonishing gentleman who had devoted his life to helping others had sadly died in such tragic circumstances at just forty-nine years old – he never did achieve his dream of retiring at 50 to become a painter.

Banting's colleagues who perished that night were named as Navigator William Bird, of Kidderminster, England and Radio Operator, William Snailham of Bedford, Nova Scotia. All three men were buried in Toronto's Mount Pleasant Cemetery. Banting received full military honours, a private service was held at the University of Toronto and his casket was flag draped on a gun carriage which paraded around the streets of Toronto. Lady Banting was presented with the Memorial Cross on her husband Major Sir Frederick Grant Banting's behalf. Once again, Banting was a war hero, this time having made the ultimate sacrifice for his country by giving his life. Banting is Toronto's hero, Canada's hero, medicines hero and a hero to everyone in the type 1 diabetes community. Banting's work is not finished, his legacy lives on. As we will see later on in this book, many people across the world do not have access to insulin, Banting's selfless "gift to mankind."

Legacy

Seven Mile Pond was later renamed Banting Lake. Captain MacKey returned to the crash site for the first time in 1971, some 30 years after the crash and paid his respects to those who perished. A memorial park is now at the site.

Sir Banting has inspired the name of several schools, colleges, university departments, hospitals, research departments, scientific centre and clinics across Canada, but also an American Liberty Ship and even a crater on the moon. The University of Toronto awards several scholarships every year in Banting's honour, to those who are interested in carrying on his scientific and medical research.

Every year, on 14th November (Banting's birthday), the diabetes community celebrates World Diabetes Day (WDD). Since 1991, this event which is organised by the International Diabetes Federation has provided an opportunity to raise awareness of the condition, collaborate and raise vital funds for charities that help people with diabetes. In 2006, the United Nations identified November 14th as an official United Nations Day. WDD is celebrated in over 160 countries and reaches out to a global audience of over 100 billion people.

The house in London, Ontario, where Banting first had his sleepless night that led to insulin development, is now named "*Banting House – the birthplace of insulin,*" and is a museum dedicated to the great man and his work. In 1991, the Queen Mother opened Banting Square just next to the house where a statue of this incredible man is now placed, she also lit a "beacon of hope" and it will only be extinguished when a true, biological cure for Type 1 Diabetes is found. The researchers who worked on the cure will be invited to extinguish the flame. The beacon gives hope to many, and until such a time comes when people can say "I used to have Type 1 Diabetes" the flame will keep on burning, an inspiration to scientists and patients alike to keep on fighting the fight against the monster that is type 1 diabetes.

In the meantime, we remain grateful to the wonderful man who had a sleepless night, genius idea and went on to discover insulin.

To find out more and to see photo's of Banting, check out our website at www.typeawesome.co.uk

Chapter 2

"I feel I was born ready to do a medical interview, because my life has been like a long medical interview!"

Jess Burton

Jess is now 20 years old and has lived with diabetes all her life. Jess has never let diabetes get in her way. In fact, after unremarkable academic achievements, she is currently studying medicine at St George's, University of London. Jess says diabetes has given her a unique perspective on life and this has benefitted her in her chosen career in medicine. Jess has an amazing story and we hope you enjoy reading it.

I was diagnosed with Congenital Hyperinsulinism (CHI) at birth. Although they didn't know it at the time, both of my parents were carriers of this genetic condition.

CHI is a genetic disorder which is quite the opposite of diabetes. Whereas people with T1D can no longer produce insulin, patients with CHI actually have a pancreas that secretes too much insulin. Excess insulin causes low plasma sugar (hypoglycaemia), or low blood sugar.

I'm sure anyone reading this is familiar with the role of insulin in the human body, but here is a very quick recap for anyone who needs it: Insulin is a hormone produced by beta cells in the pancreas. Insulin controls levels of sugar in the blood. Beta cells should release insulin in direct response to the level of glucose in the blood, so when blood glucose level is elevated the beta cells release more insulin, which allows the glucose to be absorbed from the blood. If there is a low level of glucose in the blood, such as before mealtimes, the beta cells release much smaller amounts of insulin or even turn off insulin production altogether. This keeps the blood glucose level balanced and at the right level for the rest of the human body to function normally. As well as controlling insulin release, the pancreas also secretes digestive substances called pancreatic enzymes into the first part of the small intestine (duodenum).

In patients with CHI, the beta cells release insulin inappropriately all the time, and insulin secretion is not regulated by the blood glucose level (as occurs in a normally functioning pancreas). The course of action of insulin causes the beta cells of the pancreas to release too much insulin, which in turn causes hyper-insulinaemic hypoglycemia. This effect is the same as a diabetic hypoglycaemic episode, and the patient must urgently receive the right amount of glucose in order to survive and for the body to function as it should do.

After my birth, I immediately started having multiple seizures. No one knew why at the time, so lots of tests were carried out. It was discovered that my blood sugar was low; some readings that day were as low as 0.3. It was rightly believed that this was the cause of the seizures, which still continued, so I was severely hypoglycaemic. At just 20 hours old I was placed on a glucose drip and I would remain on it for several weeks to come. I was in a constant
state of hypoglycaemia. I was officially diagnosed with Congenital Hyperinsulinism (CHI).
(Not having a pancreas does cause additional health problems that other Type 1 diabetics do not have, so I had/have other complications too, but these are not the focus of this chapter, so I will not discuss them here.)

I spent the first three months of my life in hospital. By the time I came home I had already had seven general anaesthetics and as many surgeries. A lot of different treatments for CHI were tried, (many drugs are available to try and slow down insulin secretion) but unfortunately none of them worked for me. In one of my surgeries, they removed 60% of my pancreas with the hope that they had taken away the problem cells and that the remaining ones would be able to produce the correct amount of insulin. As I came round from this surgery, it was apparent that it had not worked. I was still having seizures and getting blood sugars below 2.4, so unfortunately constant intravenous glucose was still required. Two weeks later, a further surgery was required to remove the rest of my pancreas.

The problem with removing the pancreas to resolve an excess insulin production is that there is no pancreas left at all to produce the insulin we all need to live. This, in theory, made me insulin dependent; however, I was not yet at this stage classed as Type 1 diabetic, although it was certainly in the post.

Over the next couple of weeks following the surgery, my blood sugars rose, albeit very, very slowly at first. It took two weeks for me to no longer need the glucose drip, and at six weeks old I had my very first insulin injection. I think my first insulin shot was a very minute amount as I was so small! My life was now to be shaped by diabetes, along with the insulin injections, strict regime, set meal times, and blood tests that came with it back then. Twenty years ago, there were no pen needles, and treatment focused on having very strict set mealtimes and insulin doses, which would be delivered with a proper syringe.

The early days

The first six or seven years of my life, I had a lot of hypos. My mum struggled to work whilst also managing my medical care. I was too young to take full responsibility myself, and back then schools did not legally have to provide medical treatment (this changed in 2014). My mum had to be close by to my school as they would also require support and advice, and Mum may be needed to come in and give me injections or other treatments. I also would be sent home from school a lot, or be absent for medical procedures, appointments and overnight stays in hospital. My mum adapted by working from home in my early years, as this provided her with some flexibility in which she could still care for me and help me manage my diabetes and the inevitable complications but also contribute to the household income.

A major breakthrough

Towards the later years of junior school, I was old enough to have some understanding of my condition and what I needed to do to manage it. I know my mum constantly worried about what life would have in store for me, fearing that my life revolved around medical regimes, and I know she was living in fear that hypos would prevent me from doing the things I loved.

By the age of eight or nine came a major breakthrough: I started carrying my own medical kit! Sometimes, I would even do my own testing or injections, and this new found independence gave me and Mum some reassurance that I could get on with my life. Carrying my own medical kit might seem such a small thing, but it really was a huge step towards independence for me.

At age eleven I started acting in stage shows. I was chosen to play the lead character, Amber Von Tussle, in the show Hairspray. We had to plan for every eventuality on stage. What if I had a hypo? How would I get treatment without jeopardizing the show? A hypo treatment box was kept to the left of the stage, just behind the curtain, out of sight of the audience, but in sight for me. This simple initiative meant I could continue acting, but with the reassurance that treatment was in sight if needed. Plus, I could just keep sipping the Lucozade in between scenes in order to keep my bloods up. This worked, as the majority of the time I was on stage my bloods were high, usually 20 or higher, but this meant I could get on with my life. Crazy high blood sugars meant I could do things without the fear of a hypo looming, my mum could relax in the audience knowing I would be okay, and even if I felt funny, the hypo treatments were within my reach. I went on to star in many stage shows and never had a hypo on stage.

The school trip

I was fifteen when my stage school organized a week long residential to Italy. I came home asking Mum if I could go. The price was affordable and this was a performing arts trip, but Mum could have said no. Previously, my mum had accompanied me on school trips, but she wouldn't be able to come on this one.
I was surprised that my Mum immediately said yes, I could go to Italy. Many years later I found out that Mum wanted to say no, but she knew she couldn't go back on her word. Mum had realized this was the first stage in beginning to let go. Had she said no, she would have been letting diabetes stop me from having this amazing experience. I was so pleased I could go.

The trip took months of planning. We had to think of every possible eventuality, come up with a solution to it, and then write detailed care plans. All the teachers who went on the trip had to learn extensively about diabetes, including the highs and lows, how to treat them, the effects of carbohydrates on blood sugars, how to count carbs, and how to work my medical equipment. Additional concerns were how the change in climate would affect my bloods, and how Italian foods might be different from the foods I ate at home, so there were dietary considerations. Italians love pizza and pasta!

When we got to Italy, the weather was very hot. As always happens in the heat, my blood sugars dropped, and whilst we were unpacking at the hotel, my sugars were in the twos. I remember one of the female teachers sat in the bedroom with me whilst we all unpacked our cases. This teacher was talking to us all, so that I didn't stand out as different or "sick", but I knew she was really there to keep an eye on me. I felt the teachers adapted to me, not me to them. I am still good friends with this teacher, even though I am now at university. I had an excellent week on the Italy trip, which otherwise went without incident, and it was another huge step forward with my independence. I am so grateful to Mum for letting me go. I appreciate it must have been worrying for her, but I think it put me in good stead for leaving home and going to university.

Medical School

I grew up visiting hospitals as both an outpatient and inpatient, and this clearly had an effect on me, as I always wanted to be a nurse. I could see how the nurses were on the front line and actively involved in patient care. I found this inspiring and I too wanted to make a difference to the lives of other people and help them in managing their conditions. As I grew older, I would take a lot of time at hospital to pay attention to what each medical professional was doing. I realized that while nurses play this vital role, it is the doctors who make the potentially life-changing decisions. They are the ones who study medical conditions and use their scientific knowledge to diagnose and treat, in turn improving the lives of their patients. Doctors can also undertake scientific research, which can enhance understanding and treatment of medical conditions and can even make scientific and medical breakthroughs in understanding and treatments of conditions. I decided that being a doctor is more in line with what I want to achieve, and how I can enable patients to lead their best life. I chose to study subjects that would get me into medical school, and I devoted a lot of time to make sure I got accepted!

I began to research medical school and came to the conclusion that my experiences as a patient could actually put me at an advantage. During my hospital visits, I would watch what the doctors were doing. I would ask questions and compare this to my work experience – at this time I was working in a care home to gain some experience in a clinical setting.

I remember at my interview for medical school thinking my experience as a patient allowed me to sail through the interview. One of the questions was about the technology that is involved in treating medical conditions. I immediately started talking about my insulin pump. I remember telling the interviewers that twenty years ago all people with diabetes were using injections, all patients were on the same regime of strict mealtimes and set meals, and there was no room for movement or individualised treatment plans. All individuals had exactly the same treatment plan in those days. Nowadays, an electronic pancreas is entirely possible, which means patients can have their own individualized treatment and manage diabetes using what works best for them. With advances in technology it is exciting to see where we will be in just ten years' time. I feel I was born ready to do a medical interview, because my life has been like a long medical interview!
I remember during medical training, I was part of a group of four

students. After a lot of classroom work, lectures, and academic essays, we were finally allowed on the wards for the first time. My fellow students were scared and nervous. They were staring at the clinically clean ward, anxiously looking at the patients in their beds, and were nervous about interacting with them. My colleagues were worried about what they were wearing, wondering if they were dressed right for the job. I felt differently; I was already familiar with the clinical environment, the starched white sheets and the smell of disinfectant. I was familiar with medical equipment, sharps bins, and the yellow bin bags for clinical waste. I knew that what really mattered was how we smile at patients, as my own experience has taught me that a simple smile can really change a hospital patient's day. I understand that patients need things explaining to them in a manner that they can understand. I know from my experience that the patient needs to feel listened to, and they need to feel in control of their own care. Whilst my colleagues wondered about the right shoes, I was wondering how best to connect with these individuals on the ward.

Diabetes has put me at an advantage when I am providing bedside care. I feel I can connect with patients on a different level to my colleagues as a result of my own experiences. I can certainly empathise with them. I find it very easy to be compassionate! When patients tell me that they do not like needles, I can genuinely empathise and I say, "I completely understand what you are going through".

I am twenty years old, so I still have a long way to go in medical school before I finally qualify as a doctor. I still have a lot to learn and experience before I need to decide on a specialty. I am, however, already showing a special interest in whole-of-the-body conditions. Perhaps this is influenced by my diabetes. Maybe one day I will specialize in a whole-of-body condition like diabetes, rheumatology, or paediatrics. I find these patients tend to require more complex care, as their medical diagnosis affects multiple systems in the human body. I find this interesting as a doctor because it is vital that each system is managed, and their care must be managed across multiple disciplines. I have seen how patients sometimes have to fight for a blood test or access to equipment and technology that is needed to manage their health and improve their life. I have the unique perspective of seeing both sides, and I hope I can be that person for my patients who can advocate for their best interests, not just diagnosing and treating them, but seeing the whole person.

Going to university and leaving home is a major step for anyone, but as a person with diabetes it brings additional anxieties. I have put together some tips below for young people, but I hope it also is useful to any parents who may be nervous about their child leaving home and going to university.

The rest of this chapter is adapted from my blog (link at end of chapter). I am going to explain how university works for me, maybe these tips will help you or someone you know who is going to uni and also lives with Type 1.

Tips for University

Tip #1 – Communicate with the university
Uni is leaps and bounds from school. You're comforted, supervised and guided at school, whereas uni is a much more independent and self-guided educational experience. That doesn't mean they can't help you. I emailed the disability expert at the student help centre on A-level results day (you can do this earlier if you accept a conditional offer before results day) and went from there. I ended up travelling to my uni to have a meeting with the disability officer to put together a 'care plan' (for want of a better term).

This document covered provision for exams, overnight at the student accommodation, emergency protocols, and future work placements. It has been a godsend. Exams were all in my own room with stop-the-clock/extra time arrangements allowing me to monitor my bloods and treat accordingly. I trained all of the eight resident advisors (these are older students who work for the uni by taking it in turns to live at the student accommodation, so they are there overnight) on how to use the glucagon. On my first placement this year, I contacted the student point-of-contact at the hospital who helped me arrange a disabled parking space for free for the duration of my course, and she gave me extra details (more than other students) about things like where the lockers were so I could pre-plan where I would keep my medical stuff, which ended up being on me in my pockets. This was all possible because my uni knows my name and knows I'll occasionally need extra help.

Conclusion: The disability officer will make your life easier. Make a point of meeting them and knowing them. I made sure I did all this rather than my mum (she did this role with schools), because I was the one who would need to contact them for help.

Tip #2 – Overnight arrangements

Each uni will do this differently and I can only comment on mine, but the arrangement I had in place worked for us.

My mum has my blood sugars on her phone every night and this alerts her if I'm dropping or rising. If I am low for say one hour or reach 3.0mmol/l, my mum will ring me. If I don't answer my mobile she calls the security desk at the student halls (my halls of residence has a receptionist during the daytimes and 24-hour security guards at the front desk) who will phone my room phone or put her through to me on the room phone to sort me out. Each room has a phone in it (an old fashioned one) that was significantly more jarring than my ring tone, so I would more often than not wake up to this. On two or three occasions my mum would ask them to go to my room or the security guard would decide that, and he would call the RA (Resident Advisor) for that night. Then the two of them would come and let themselves in (thankfully knocking beforehand). If I needed an ambulance they would've called one, and the RA was glucagon trained. This worked well for me. Although, it can be a bit of a shock to wake up at 4 a.m. to a loud voice proclaiming 'Miss Burton, we're coming in!'

Conclusion: Don't say no to help with overnights just because you want to be independent as you move out. You'll already be tired from the lifestyle shock and brain-frying lectures. You need your sleep. Let other people help you overnight and also have others be your back up.

Tip #3 – GP and pharmacy shenanigans

I told my GP's surgery at home that I was moving to uni and I was told that I would have to register with a GP there. Well that scuppered my plans completely. I'd been advised that it was a good idea to stay with my home GP, because they know you, for getting prescriptions and also for having appointments in holiday times as you do spend a lot of time at home, even if you're a uni student. Well before I knew it, I'd registered with a GP around the corner from my uni and was thrown into a completely new routine with them.

Don't get me wrong, I am pleased with my decision in the end. I like having my GP near uni and that it gives me independence in this area of my medical life that I didn't seek before. It also forces me to be on top of my other non-diabetes needs, appointments and prescriptions. I also don't need to wait to get appointments in holidays, as studying medicine you don't get as many holidays as some other courses, especially as I get to 3rd year and beyond.

However, it hasn't been without its problems. Initially I struggled to get along with my GP as she was very by-the-book and even though she was a lovely person and addressed all my needs in my appointments and checked/prescribed whatever I needed, I found

that she needed a letter from my endocrinologist for every prescription change, she wanted me to book double appointments and seemed to get exasperated when I didn't (I didn't because I hadn't deemed my issue double-appointment worthy). She did though. I also messed up my prescription the first time and had to get emergency meds as I hadn't put in an order. That has happened twice now, and I'm sure my pharmacy think I'm not on top of it half the time.

Saying all of that, I'm now on top of it all. I know what I have in stock, when I need it, and I feel independent with this side of things.

Conclusion: Plan ahead what you're going to do about GP and pharmacy. Don't fall into something you don't want to do like I did, but do consider all options because the option I fell into worked well for me after all.

Tip #5 (a token non-diabetes tip) – Budget, budget, budget.
Money. The thing EVERYONE wants to talk about, right? Not. Even better to talk about: students' money. Or lack thereof.

When it comes to money at uni I have only one tip: budget. It is especially important to budget when you are living with diabetes, because you do not want to run out of money for food. You never know when you will need to buy a hypo treatment. If you forget to take in a sandwich you will need to buy lunch in the canteen, and you just might need money for transport to get to appointments or other places you go to for support.

Be realistic about your budget though.

1. Don't leave yourself £10 a week for food. I spend between £25 and £50 a week on food, sometimes a little more if I've eaten out that week. I get my Lidl shopping but I also forget to pack myself lunch a lot of days, so there's extra money out of my account. You could skip buying lunch, sure. Some of my friends do that to maintain their budget, but as a person with diabetes when you're sat in your 2 p.m. lecture at a 3.1mmol/l, you'll regret that tiny £10 food budget that took your emergency lunch money away.

2. Are you really only going to spend £20 on drinks on a night out? No. You're a student. Probably in a big city. Nightclub drinks are expensive. Even if you don't drink when you're out and instead do pre-drinks to get drunk before heading out, that £20 Smirnoff came out of your account. Then don't forget to add the two cartons of orange juice you bought as mixers. They won't have cost you a lot but it takes you over the possible budget you set. Girls, you'll probably have bought a new outfit or a new lipstick for the evening. Who bought the pre-drinks games? It all adds up. If that's what you want to spend your money on, go for it! Just allow for that in your budgeting.

3. Extras. Don't assume you'll go the whole year without going clothes shopping once, funding your hobby or needing to pay a society fee. It happens. So leave a little surplus money each week or each month that can be used for all the unexpected fun.

4. Prioritise your budget. Don't allow £100 a week for alcohol and nights out but only allow £5 a week for stationery. You are, after all, at uni. Its primary goal is to get you a degree, so some money for that is a good idea. Plus, don't forget travel. Public transport is a lot of money so don't spend your last £10 of the week on that new top. What if on Friday you sleep badly so need to get the bus in the morning instead of walking? What if you wake up on a 3.6mmol/l?

Conclusion: Note it down. Properly think about it. Can you afford whatever you're holding? I used an app to record my spending for the first month or so, which helped give me an idea of what I was spending so then I could refine my budget.

Tip #5 – Don't panic.

Uni is fun. It is scary, for everyone, but first and foremost it's fun. I realise everyone has different uni experiences and I can, again, only comment on my own, but I firmly believe you make your own uni experience.

Conclusion: No matter how you're feeling, everything will be okay. If you're feeling lonely go and chat to someone, because the chances are they're feeling lonely too. You'll need to solve your own issues with this kind of stuff now, but everyone else does too.

My last advice is this: it's important that you go to freshers' fayre, walk up to that group of people you heard talking about your favourite show, and if your flat mates invite you out, go with them (if they don't invite you, maybe it's your job to invite them this time). Stay up until 5 a.m. chatting with people who will be strangers at the moment, because soon they're the people keeping you sane during the year. Sign up for that random society, explore the student bar, and muster up the courage to just say yes. Eat utter garbage, mess up your diet or exercise, and get lost wandering corridors. Things will undoubtedly go wrong and not go to plan. That's okay. Branch out. Go with the flow. Uni is scary, uni is fun, and it is certainly a wild ride. Just roll with it. You'll be thankful you did.

This one is very important: be yourself. Not always the easiest thing, but it's seriously the best way to get the friends you're meant to be with.

But the most important thing of all?

Have fun!

It's the perfect place to do just that.

Oh and don't forget to test along the way (I guess that's important too…)!

Jess' tip for parents of a child with diabetes: don't ask your child about their blood sugars as soon as they come in from school, ask them how they are first, ask how their day went and if they had fun before asking about bloods.

Jess's tip for a young person with diabetes: Test! Don't beat yourself up if you have a bad day. Just do what you need to do and ask for help if needed.

Jess has a blog "Pancreasless and Proud" where she blogs about health, medical school and the ups and downs of blood sugars.

https://pancreasless.wordpress.com/

To find out more about Jess and to see pictures of her in "scrubs" and proudly displaying her CGM at prom, check out our website at **www.typeawesome.co.uk**

Chapter 3

"The Sky Really is the Limit!"

Glen Freeman

Glen is 39 and lives in London, England. Glen was diagnosed at just 18 months old so does not remember a time when he lived without diabetes. Glen has a fantastic attitude towards his diabetes, he has not let it stop him from doing anything in his life and he has worked hard to achieve all of his dreams, even managing to fly planes. When Glen was told he could not pilot planes, he wasn't going to take no for an answer! Glen tells us all about his life with diabetes and has some great advice that he wants to share.

I was diagnosed at just 18 months old, so I have no memory of diagnosis but from what I am told, I displayed the usual symptoms of insatiable thirst, more wet nappies than usual, increased tiredness and weight loss. I have no recollection of life without diabetes, which I think it actually a good thing as it normalizes everything for me. I think this is probably why I believe it is completely normal to test, inject and carb count every time I want to eat or drink (and of course, at other times too). I don't see myself as any different from a person without diabetes, just I have to take extra care of myself at times. Sometimes taking care of myself involves a lot more input and certainly a lot more invasive procedures than my friends without diabetes require, but I have come to accept it is normal for me and it is just something I have to do. Sure, I do get fed up of diabetes at times, of course, this condition is relentless and never gives me a break, but letting it stop me or giving in to it would be letting it win. One thing for sure, diabetes will never win or take over my life, sometimes I see it as a game and I am a poor loser at this game.

I grew up in Cornwall, a beautiful county in South West England. Cornwall is a stunningly beautiful county, its south coast is referred to as the Cornish Riviera and it boasts hundreds of Sandy beaches, picturesque harbour villages, whilst the north coast has rugged cliffs and great surfing close by. The inland areas of Cornwall have wild moorlands and Dartmoor, one of England's 10 National Parks, is just over the county boundary in Devon. Cornwall is an idyllic place to grow up and it influenced my hobbies and activities I took part in when I was growing up.

I have fond memories of my first Paediatric Diabetes Specialist Nurse (PDSN), Patsy, she was lovely and very supportive, as I am sure your diabetes nurse is too. Patsy helped me see that diabetes does not define me, she would tell me that I am not diabetic, but I am a person. A person living with diabetes. Something about what Patsy said stuck with me and I have always kept this to the front of my mind and used it as an inspiration. I feel that in my adult life, I have Patsy and her wise words in my diabetes toolkit, giving me advice and the courage to carry on.

I have always had insulin injections, when I was young there was no alternative. Back in the early 1980's the technology that was used to manage diabetes was very different when compared to the technology used today. My syringes had massive plastic plungers with long scary needles. Management was different too, I had very strict meal times and a set number of injections at a certain time each day, this didn't give me the freedom that I have now to eat and drink what and when I want. Fast acting insulin (Novorapid) is a fantastic invention and certainly allows more freedom, flexibility and choice around mealtimes.

Diabetes did not define me, although the injections were important, I was just a boy getting on with my life. I fondly recall just being a boy, getting muddy and playing roly poly down the hills in my local park. I loved playing in the sand on Cornwall's stunning beaches. When you think of a Cornish beach, you are probably imagining an ice cream. My childhood certainly contained a lot of ice cream. In fact, selling ice cream was my first job as a teenager!

During my teenage years, maybe around age 14 or 15 I started showing an interest in aircraft and flying. I would watch the military planes in training flights over RAF St Mawgan, a Royal Air Force base in Newquay, Cornwall. I was fascinated with the planes, I learnt a lot about them, could recite facts about them and could often be found just watching them on training. I also used to look at larger jets taking people to and from their holidays and dream about the different places they had been. On family holidays abroad, whilst I was on the plane I would dream of being in the cockpit myself piloting the plane and taking people all around the world. What a fantastic job that would be! One day I wanted to be a pilot myself. I wanted to get in the cockpit.

I was told that flying a plane with Type 1 diabetes was not possible. Certainly, in those days it was a job on the barring list, so any person who lives with type 1 diabetes, like myself, could not fly planes or get a pilot's license. As there currently is no cure for Type 1 Diabetes, I was told that my dream of flying a plane would have to be over.

I did not accept this. I was fine flying around the world as a passenger and would put my insulin and any other supplies in a bag that I kept with me throughout the flight. In order to manage my diabetes, I would test on the plane and give myself insulin or sugar accordingly in order to properly manage my condition. Why couldn't I do this if I was a Pilot? And I would have a co-pilot if there was an emergency. I did not take no for an answer, so I joined my local Air Cadet Squadron!

Air Cadets was amazing. I was treated just the same as everyone else, that is because I was the same as everyone else. I gained a lot of independence and confidence there and those skills are still used to this day. Air Cadets got really exciting, especially when we went away to real air bases on camps at weekends and school holidays. At these camps, we joined in fully with life on the air base and amazingly that included flying. As everyone is treated as equal within the Air Training Corps, my diabetes did not bar me from flying! Type 1 Diabetes is not a condition that bars a person from flying with the Air Cadets, as long as they take extra precautions, such as testing their bloods beforehand, having immediate access to hypo treatments and following the other rules. Imagine how good I felt when I was behind the cockpit of a Chipmunk for the first time, an exciting moment for anybody but after previously being told I could not fly it felt like I could do anything at all!

I also did 2-day walks with the Air Cadets across the hills of Dartmoor. The potential problem here was of course the risk of going hypo whilst on the top of the hills. Dartmoor would be a difficult place to get emergency services to and it would almost certainly involve the Mountain Rescue! It was therefore vital that I took with me everything that I might possibly need, I had to plan for every eventuality as if it was certain to happen. That way, I would have whatever I needed with me if the eventuality occurred. Of course, taking part in these two day walks   just took a little more planning than it would have done for a person living without diabetes. I also had more equipment to carry, not just extra testing strips, batteries for the blood glucose meter, insulin pens, needles but food, hypo treatments, long acting carbohydrate snacks to keep my blood up. All this was much more important to me than my peers, but it was a small price to pay in return for the amazing feeling I got when I reached the peak of each tor of Dartmoor. I felt elated at every summit and I have used this same can-do attitude throughout my adult life when I stumble across hurdles, whether they are diabetes related or not. Many things in life just involve planning for all eventualities and the motivation to act.

I was 18 when I left home and went to University. I attended Brunel University in West London and I studied E-Commerce, graduating with a 2:1 Honours Degree. I lived on campus and fully participated in campus life. I can't think of one thing diabetes stopped me doing during my student years, I went out and joined in with the clubs & societies, made some life-long friends and certainly took advantage of the student union bar. It was fantastic to be living in London, where I still live and I took full advantage of everything that living in the capital had to offer.

Of course, sometimes I had hypo's and needed to treat myself, or I needed to take care of my blood sugars during exams, but University for me was successful both academically and socially. Universities are good at supporting students. Mentioning my diabetes, I was given a large room, with its own fridge, one of the closest to the centre of the university. They offered Extra time during exams, this is because I may need to test or treat hypo's, the time it takes to do this (and recover from a hypo because of course, you would not be cognitively aware when bloods are low so would be unfairly disadvantaged during exams) is not counted as exam time and they can add this onto the time at the end. You can also arrange to take your exam in a separate room to everyone else, this is useful if you are worried about your pump or CGM alarming and disrupting others. The university also had its own medical centre where I was a well-known visitor. They took great care of me.

Many of my friends at University didn't realise that I live with diabetes, it wasn't because I didn't want to tell them, it was just never really an issue to me or them and I did all the things they did. If we ate out, or I got a new housemate, they would wonder what I was doing when I got my testing kit or an insulin pen out, so I simply told them that I live with diabetes. It wasn't a problem to them, they just let me get on with treating myself without judgement. I did however have to educate them on the importance of them not eating my snacks, but overall, they were very supportive.

After University I had several jobs in the travel and finance industries. I even designed online booking systems for airlines, keeping my links to aeroplanes. I passed my driving test and used to drive to and from work every day. Diabetes was never a problem for me with my driving.

After a few years of working I decided to take a career break. My initial plan was to travel and end up in Australia, where I intended to work. I had a stop-over in China on the way out and I loved it, it was my first time in China, although not my first time in the Far East. When I got to Australia, I found it really hard to find work, it was a real challenge to keep going and support myself financially. Bizarrely, through people I met in China on the stop-over on the way out, I was offered a job in China teaching English! I accepted it immediately, applied for my visa in Brisbane, I hopped on a plane and arrived in China very excited about this amazing opportunity that lay ahead of me.

I learnt a lot about the Chinese culture, it was hard not to as I was so immersed in it. Everything is different in China; the people, the food, the school system, social norms, landscapes, the bustling cities and even walking down the street was an assault on the senses. I had arrived in Dongguan, Guangdong Province, I hired a local estate agent to help me find a flat, I found a job and had the correct work permits. I also had a good supply of insulin to last me a while, so I did not have to worry too much about that until after I had settled in. When insulin supplies did start getting low, at first, I would re-stock by flying home to visit family and get my supplies in the UK and take them back to China. Eventually, I met an international Doctor, he helped me obtain insulin without having to fly back to England every time. He was able to prescribe me everything I needed and he sourced it from Hong Kong. Although it was very expensive, about £100 for a month's supply of Novorapid disposable pens, it was worth it. I also knew that if I needed anything, he was available to see me and help me sort any medical difficulties, although thankfully, I didn't have any emergencies or need any additional diabetes care whilst I lived in China.

I very much enjoyed China, I worked in a variety of organisations teaching English to Chinese young people, my roles were varied and ranged from teaching English to children in Government schools, teaching in private schools and even in a technical college, which was really awesome. I interacted with my students and their families outside of work and they were very keen to show me around and take me to the places tourists don't find. I was grateful for these experiences and many even invited me to their homes. I was learning Mandarin Chinese and found the language fascinating, I would practice with my students and you could say that they taught me more than I taught them. It was a whole new way of life.

Living and working in China enlightened my life. I highly recommend everyone travels and has experiences in different
cultures. I fully immersed myself in the Chinese lifestyle and am so

pleased I did. Diabetes was never really an issue except on one occasion where a Chinese teacher said *"You are disabled, why don't you stay at home and not work?"* after I had a hypo in school. I got to share with her how different things are in the UK. That the government provides insulin and people lead happy normal lives. I did find at first that I had more hypo's than usual, but this was mainly because the diet is very different over there. I had to try different foods and learn about how they affected my body, then adjust insulin levels the next time I had the same food. Chinese diets are very different to the one we have in the UK and many foods I was used to weren't available. Chinese food in China is much less sugary than Chinese food in the UK. We travel to have new experiences after all and I had to find a way for diabetes to fit into my new life in China.

I eventually came back to England to continue my career. I continued to learn Mandarin and to immerse myself in the Chinese culture. In London, I continued practicing Mandarin and integrating myself into the Chinese community there, I met a wonderful young lady called Mengting. Mengting helped me to practice my Mandarin, we got on so well and she eventually became my girlfriend, the rest they say is history. Seven years on and we are still happy together. I am involved in the Chinese community in London, I work with Chinese people to help them achieve their dreams. I work with both the Chinese who are visiting London or are here for University or work, as well as Chinese people who were born here and have lived in London all their lives. I love helping people reach their goals, I am a coach and a mentor for them and I hope I can help them get the most out of their life and hope I can be as welcoming and hospitable to them as they were to me during my time in China.

I have had a successful career and quite a few different jobs. My diabetes has never got in the way of my career or been a problem in any job I have had. I wouldn't let it do that. I am just the same as my colleagues who do not live with diabetes and I am treated as so. If you do need any "reasonable adjustments" making (under the Equality Act, 2010), employers have the legal duty to provide this. Examples of reasonable adjustments in employment for people living with diabetes could include:

- Having to take time out to test, but this time could be added onto the end of the working day
- Being allowed to have a sugary drink during work to keep bloods up
- Slight adjustments to lunch time might be needed in order to avoid hypo, if the working environment does not already allow this flexibility
- Time off for appointments, tests and treatment for diabetes related issues (if these cannot be arranged for outside working hours)
- Not driving or operating machinery when recovering from a hypo, of course, it would be very dangerous if they expected you to do so
- Provide a safe place to inject – they cannot ask you to do this in the toilet for example, as it is not hygienic. I have always just done my injections where ever I happen to be, although I do try to be discreet out of respect for others.

I have always managed to fit diabetes management around me and my working day, I don't fit my working day around diabetes. I find this very easy to do these days because I am now self-employed and work to my own schedule.

I am excited about technology and I built myself a successful career working for and consulting with companies in the field of computer data. I now have my own companies, one is Property Data Engine, which focuses on helping property founders launch and grow businesses with the right processes, systems and data. My other company is Response Accommodation, which is helping heads of housing support key-workers and vulnerable people by supplying much needed safe accommodation.

I am analytical and enjoy working with data, when I think back over my years of living with Type 1 Diabetes, I can see how technology and data has improved management and treatment options. Data can inform treatment, improve management and encourage better health. Better health today prevents the long-term problems that diabetes can cause, like kidney problems, blindness, foot problems and so on. It is now possible to download the data from a pump or Continuous Glucose Monitor (CGM), these can allow you to see patterns and adjust, this was just not possible years ago when I was diagnosed. Spotting these patterns provides the opportunity to adjust insulin doses and results in better management, less hypo's and highs so more time "in range" and overall better control. It is even possible now for the data to automatically feed into a computer and communicate with clinic without the user having to do anything. Of course, the real advantage of technology and data is a CGM having the ability to communicate with a pump and make automatic adjustments to insulin doses, taking away the need for the user to interact with the technology as much. It is a very exciting time to see the developments in technology, JDRF have some exciting projects they are funding and I can see that a cure is now possible during my lifetime. I can't wait for the day I can say "I used to live with diabetes."

I now wear a Freestyle Libre flash glucose monitor alongside a Miao Miao, and I can use my phone and even my watch to check my glucose levels – how different is this to the technology of the 1980's, with a plastic plunger or a scary, painful 1990's lancet device to prick the finger to draw blood! Compare todays modern technology with 35 - 40 years ago when sugar levels were tested by urine sticks, the advancement is unbelievable. Urine testing wasn't an accurate way to test the sugar levels, it just wasn't possible to know the exact amount of sugar that was present, urine sticks basically told you if you were hypo or hyper. Also, the urine could have been in the body for several hours, which meant the sugar levels being tested could also be hours old. Clinical decisions were being made based on samples that were hours old! Now we have the ability to take an accurate reading in a flash.

The first early blood glucose meters would be the size of brick, so heavy to carry around and they would take several minutes to read the blood sample – again not good when you are a young boy waiting to see if you are hypo and need some sugar, or wondering whether diabetes is just playing you up, or maybe you feel a bit unwell for another reason. These days, I can simply look at my watch and know what my blood sugar level is at that precise moment. Amazing!

It is really inspiring to think that a technological "cure" is just around the corner. It would be fantastic to wear a device that does everything, a pump communicating with a CGM and automatically calculating the amount of insulin needed. I am currently looking forward to my first insulin pump.

Diabetes has not impacted my life whatsoever, I am just a person. I just also happen to live with diabetes. The sky really is the limit!

My advice is to get out there and do whatever you want to do, diabetes gives you more to think about but definitely should not hinder your life choices.

My advice to parents is to trust your child, allow them to take control even if they are getting it a bit wrong as they can only be independent and learn when you start letting go.

To connect with Glen go to
https://www.linkedin.com/in/knowledgeinvestor/ or
https://www.facebook.com/PropertyAndTravelTechnologist

Glen's property business is www.propertydataengine.com
Glen's supportive housing business is **www.responseaccommodation.com**

To find out more about Glen and to see photo's of him in the cockpit, check out our website at **www.typeawesome.co.uk**

Chapter 4

"Diabetes isn't a barrier, just a hurdle we have to leap over. Sometimes, we have to leap over a lot, but we can still leap"

Jade Byrne

Jade is an actress, writer and author, she has lived with T1 for thirty-one years. Jade started her career in theatre and moved onto TV roles in Casualty, Inspector George Gently, The Dumping Ground and Mount Pleasant. More recently, Jade wrote her own theatre piece, a one woman play comically named "Pricks" which has sold out at the Edinburgh Fringe Festival and then toured extensively around the United Kingdom. Jade also has an Etsy shop, selling comical T1 kit bags, hoodies etc along with her children's book Daisy Donald, a story about a girl who's a superhero in her own right as she comes with Type 1 Diabetes each day, it brings comfort and understanding to others who either have Type 1 or love someone with Type 1. It's also been used in schools to educate classes and help them learn what their classmate or teacher has to deal with each day.

I have lived with Type 1 Diabetes for 31 years, I was diagnosed on Monday 6th November, 1989. I was four years old. My earliest memories are hiding from doctors and nurses because I didn't want them to prick me. I used to hide under the hospital bed or in the wardrobe and my parents would play along pretending they didn't know where I was, but this one time I somehow got out of the hospital room and I hid behind a bin in the medicine room on the ward. In 1989 these rooms didn't have locks on them. I hid for over 2 hours apparently. I distinctly remember peering over the top of the bin and watching my family with doctors and nurses frantically calling my name walking up and down the corridor past the door. I thought it was hilarious at the time and I am still the best person in the world at hide and seek even now at 35 years old.

Back in the late 1980's, diabetes equipment was a little pre-historic, if Fred Flintstone had been diabetic, he would have used the sort of equipment I was given after my diagnosis. The blood glucose meter was massive, it took an eternity to take a reading and the finger pricker device itself was like a medieval torture device. I am most pleased that finger prickers and lancets are much gentler these days, if they need to be used at all (as alternatives are now available – I now use a Dexcom G6). I had 2 injections a day, as an adult it was increased to 4 injections a day. Very strict meal times had to be adhered to, I was quite pleased when I made the change to MDI (Multi Daily Injections) because it gave me a lot more freedom around what and when I ate. MDI and fast acting insulin made my life easier.

I was a very active teenager, interested in dancing, drama, performing arts and acting. I went into sixth form and then drama school. I would literally be dancing for 12 hours a day every day. Of course, this was great for my career and fitness, but not for the hypo's it induces!

I didn't want my tutors or people I was working with to know if my blood sugar was low because I was afraid they'd see it as my weakness. I didn't tell people as I thought I'd lose my solos or parts

I'd worked hard for. They all knew I had Type 1 Diabetes but I just didn't want people to know if I was hypo, instead, I would treat it without drawing attention to it, this almost backfired completely once though. I was near to collapsing in a rehearsal for the show Apples, which was my first big theatre tour I did. I'd been rehearsing this one scene with only me in it over and over again for maybe an hour or 2 and I knew my blood sugar was low but I did not want the director to know. I did not want my diabetes monster to defeat me. The director realised something was wrong in the end and I admitted I thought my blood sugar was low, he was totally understanding and sent me to sort it out, it was actually 1.6 when I tested, no wonder they were making me repeat the scene over and over again, I must have been doing an awful job at 1.6.

When I'm performing in theatre I always have hypo treatment backstage or in the case of Pricks, there's a secret drawer in my set with Apple Juice cartons in it. To be honest, I've never needed it though, the adrenaline does the opposite and makes my blood sugar go high. It is much easier to manage these days, I am currently on an Omnipod Dash pump and I can put a temporary basal (background insulin) on to reduce the highs whilst performing. I usually run a temp basal of plus 35% whilst I'm performing Pricks.

One of my favourite jobs ever was the filming for Inspector George Gently, I really enjoyed everything about this production – the role I played, my fellow actors, the crew, the set and the production company. I remember my first day filming, being in a posh people carrier in preparation to be moved around the set, there were 3 of us actors waiting to set off, myself, Kate Bracken and Vincent Regan. I had my bag with me and Kate said to me "Oh, you've brought a bag with you?" I replied "Yes, I have Type 1 diabetes and it's got my Lucozade and blood tester in" Kate pulled out some Dextrose tablets from her bra and replied, "Me too, I'm Type 1 diabetic." Kate was the first person I ever spent considerable time with who also had

Type 1 Diabetes, this was 22 years after my diagnosis! This was my first TV job and the other guest lead was also Type 1! It was the best 3 weeks filming ever.

One year when I was at the Edinburgh Fringe Festival, I was there as part of my job to scout for new shows for us to programme. I was inspired by many of the acts I saw, so inspired that I was sitting in the Gilded Balloon bar, as you do at the Fringe and I had a glass of wine. Over this glass of wine, the idea for my play "Pricks" was born. I had really wanted to make my own piece of theatre for a while at this point, I wanted to write a 2 hander (having seen a lot of one man shows that year I was sick on one man shows). I started brainstorming ideas, thinking of subjects I am passionate about, subjects that I know a lot about and subjects with a range of emotions involved. As I was writing some ideas down, I felt a hypo come on. As I was treating the hypo, I had a bit of a light bulb moment; something went "ping" inside of my head. I had my subject, there it was - it hit me like the sugar hit my hypo - I would write a show about living with diabetes. I would write a show to educate people about diabetes in a fun way. I certainly knew a lot about living with diabetes, it involves a range of emotions and it seemed a great way to raise awareness, which is something I am passionate about.

Initially, I was going to call the play "75,000 Pricks and counting" as that is how many injections & finger pricks I estimated I had had at that point, but I decided to shorten it to just "Pricks", let's face it, it's a much better title. When I started writing it wasn't a two hander that naturally came out, in fact it was a one woman show, which wasn't what I thought I wanted. I ended up writing the show based on my life with Type 1 and all based on the truth as I believe this is the most honest and integrous way to tell a story. Whilst researching the play, I interviewed over 40 people who either had diabetes themselves or were a parent of a child with diabetes. I did this because I didn't want Pricks to just become my own story, I wanted it to be inclusive for everyone else who lives with diabetes and for the show to tell their stories also. Diabetes is different in everyone, we all have different symptoms for highs and lows, different triggers for hypers and hypos, we all have different experiences in school and the workplace with managing our diabetes and these days we all certainly have different treatment options available. I needed to make sure I told my story and it was clear it was my story, but that it included bits of everyone else too whilst still making it accessible to people who don't understand Type 1 Diabetes at all, because ultimately, I wanted to educate through entertainment.

Pricks does feature other people's stories through sound bites, such as the story of Rosie who has a Dad with Type 1 and also the account of my own Mum, my Dad and my husband James. The show takes the viewer through a range of emotions – just like diabetes does! It does get quite emotional at times but you will also laugh out loud too. It takes a light hearted look of diabetes and of course, I have a whole scene dedicated to the stupid comments and questions myself and others have heard from non-type 1's, you know, the ones along the lines of "did you eat too many sweets when you were younger?" or "did you used to be fat?" and "should you be eating that?", my go to response to that last one is, "would I be eating it if I couldn't?"

Pricks debut performance was at the Durham Gala Theatre on June 8th, 2018, I also took it to Alphabetti Theatre in Newcastle and Jabberwocky Market in Darlington on the preview tour. Then it returned back to where the idea for it was first born: The Edinburgh Fringe Festival.

I admit, I was a bit nervous at first about how the show would be received. Although the preview tour had gone spectacularly well, I was still worried about the press and the what the reviewers would say. I was also concerned people would think it was self-indulgent, because really, I am the inspiration behind the show although it really is not a self-indulgent piece, which thankfully the reviews echoed. I had no need to worry as the show sold out on many days and it was a roaring success! People in the audience were laughing, but also crying as it is a very emotional show. People living without diabetes came in not knowing anything about type 1 and came out knowing much more than they could have learnt in any lecture. People with diabetes could identify and understand the range of emotions on a different level, they learnt from it too as they would see diabetes from other people's perspectives and experiences. Overall, people were gripped, every prick of the way!

As you may have gathered Edinburgh turned out to be very successful for me, the show went down well and I had succeeded in educating people through the medium of entertainment. I was now ready to take the show on the road and because of the Edinburgh platform the bookings were flying in. I did a Northern tour taking in all the areas of Yorkshire and also Manchester. It paid off, the show challenged the misconceptions and misunderstanding of type 1 diabetes in the media. I knew this because the media had started picking up on it, so by this time there was a real buzz around the show and bookings were flying in for Spring/Summer 2019 and Autumn 2019 too.

Professor Partha Kar, the NHS England lead for Diabetes, had heard about my show, in fact it had been on his radar before I'd even finished writing it and he trusted and believed in me enough to help me to get the funding from a pharmaceutical company for my Edinburgh run. Partha is also the co-creator of TAD Talks (Talking About Diabetes), which aim to bring together inspirational people who are living with diabetes. The main goal of TAD Talks is to inspire people to think differently about their condition, remove barriers and to learn about and embrace new technologies. Partha offered me the amazing opportunity to stand on stage and headline the TAD Talk 2019 with Pricks.

TAD Talk was an amazing event; many people with T1 came together and had lots of opportunities to share our experiences. It was a star-studded affair, the actor James Norton was there as he too has Type 1, he was very friendly and supportive towards me. There was a great sadness that overhung me though, unfortunately, my guardian angel as I describe her in Pricks, my Mum, was diagnosed with Acute Myeloid Leukaemia during my Autumn 2018 tour and the few months that had preceded TAD Talk were the worst of my life. Watching the person who's kept you alive and revived you from hundreds of hypos, who's held your hand through everything in life, suffer the way she did, was simply unfair. She lost her battle with Leukaemia just 6 days before the event. Knowing my Mum would have been so annoyed if I had cancelled, I went ahead despite feeling pain so raw and so deep. The show must go on has always been my motto and I am really pleased it did. 300 people in one room all connected to Type 1 Diabetes, my most feared audience, the most critical audience, they all stood on their feet at the end and applauded. That's when I knew, I truly knew, that Pricks was everything I had wanted it to be.

My Mum's death inspired me to go ahead with another venture that had been at the back of my mind for a while. I was going to write a children's book for Type 1s and anyone that needed educating about it. I'd lost the person in my life that always supported me, always drilled it into me that having Type 1 Diabetes was never going to stop me from doing anything and those messages and empowerment my Mum had always given me, needed to be shared.

Daisy Donald is the main character of my children's book, I love alliteration. I run Pricks Products (diabetes merchandise you should definitely check out on Etsy), Platform Perform, Mature Movers. Seriously can't get enough of alliteration so she had to be Daisy Donald. Daisy has superpowers and fights a monster, the monster being Type 1 Diabetes and Daisy's superpower being her resilience and strength which is needed to fight it. The aim of the book was to educate anyone who wants to read it, but ultimately emotionally support any child with Type 1 and it is especially useful to children who have just been diagnosed. Daisy Donald helps children to feel uplifted and inspired by Daisy. The book does not shy away from the lows that can be experienced by children with diabetes, but it encourages them to find strength and resilience when dealing with their own monster on a day to day basis.

From another perspective, Daisy Donald allows me to address the misunderstandings that surround this condition. I can address the younger generation as one day they will be the adults, I can challenge the myths and raise awareness and understanding. I remember saying to Partha Kar I've written this book because if we're going to change the world's perspective on Type 1 Diabetes it's best to start from the bottom up and educate people properly whilst they're young so that they can impart their wisdom for generations to come.

I had to do this for the younger Type 1s because my Mum was fantastic, she made my life as easy as it could be, she would educate people and go into school to ensure they knew everything they needed to know. I needed to know that every young Type 1 had an opportunity to have a little piece of my Mum. Many of the things my Mum used to say to me are reflected back in the book. My Mum would often tell me that I am a little bit different to everyone else, but that is really cool like a superpower. I want other children to feel special with their superpower, even though it is relentless, but hopefully by reading Daisy Donald they can feel like my Mum used to make me feel. I'm sure my Mum's amazing emotional support has made a lot of difference to my life, my career, opportunities and my future prospects.

The book is my tribute to Mum. Everything I do is a tribute to her.

I honestly think diabetes has made me the determined, strong and resilient person I am today. Daisy Donald inspires young children and shows them that they too are resilient, they are superheroes and diabetes will not stop them doing anything they want to do. Diabetes isn't a barrier, it's a hurdle we have to leap over. Sometimes we have to leap over a lot of them, but we will always continue to leap.

Jades one piece of advice to parents: Let them eat the cake!
Jades one piece of advice to people with diabetes: put on your invisible cloak and reach for the stars

Find out more about Pricks: The Play and keep up to date at:
www.prickstheplay.co.uk

Jade can also be found on all social media using @PricksOfficial

Daisy Donald can be purchased in Jade's Etsy shop, along with other fun diabetes related products:
https://www.etsy.com/uk/shop/PricksProducts?ref=l2-shop-info-avatar&listing_id=752459137

To find out more about Jade and to see photo's, check out **www.typeawesome.co.uk**

Chapter 5

"Diabetes spurred me on, it was a big setback, but one I wanted to overcome."

Jordan Thompson

Jordan is a young professional cricket player for Yorkshire County Cricket Club (YCCC), he is now 24 years old and was diagnosed with Type 1 Diabetes 9 years ago when he was 16. All Jordan ever wanted to do was be a professional sportsman and he initially worried that diabetes meant the end to his career before he had even started playing at a professional level. Jordan tells us about his diabetes and how he manages it to enable him to not only play the sport he loves, but how he rose to be at the top of his game, despite the additional challenges he can sometimes face.

I first started playing cricket as a toddler, some of my earliest memories are of playing cricket with my Dad in the garden. As a toddler, Dad would take me a long to his Cricket Club, I would love to try join in and I took an interest in the sport from an early age. In fact, I can not remember a time in my life that I didn't love cricket. Dad would have the cricket players at his club bowl to me and I would practice my batting, even though I could only just walk.

As young as 6 years old I was playing in teams, I am from Yeadon, a small town just outside Leeds, close to the airport. I played in the Yorkshire Schoolboys under nines, then when I reached 9 years old I played in the under 11s.

A local team called Pudsey St. Lawrence is where I did a lot of my childhood training and I played in many competitive matches when growing up, depending on my age and ability at the time. I was proud to represent my county, I am a proud Yorkshireman at heart and it was good to play for the Yorkshire youth team.

Even at school, my favourite subjects were the ones involving sport and fitness, I joined in all the extra-curricular activities that involved team sports and keeping fit. I am also a big football supporter, I am a Leeds United fan and try to get to the games both at home and away, when it doesn't clash with my cricket or more recently covid of course!

I live and breathe sport and I cannot remember a time when I didn't want to be a professional sportsman, especially a cricket player. I could not ever imagine doing anything else for a job other than sport. My childhood dream was to play Cricket for a living. I achieved this dream, but it wasn't without a big adversity I had to learn how to overcome.

I was 16 when I started with symptoms of Type 1 Diabetes, although I did not know what the symptoms were at the time. I was still in high school, although it was the sixth form at that stage so more like a college.

I was playing in the Yorkshire Cricket 2nd team at the time and had an intense training schedule. I can remember one particular match I was playing for the Yorkshires 2nd XI against Middlesex. My eyesight had gone blurry, I couldn't visually focus on the game or pay my attention to it as I was so tired. I kept falling asleep on the side-lines and just couldn't stay awake for the match, I felt like my eyes needed propping open with matchsticks.

I can also remember that I had lost a lot of weight, playing professional sports involves having to record these sorts of stats regularly, the weight had been dropping off me for weeks. I couldn't stop going off to the toilet, but I was also drinking a lot to stay hydrated throughout the game and although I have always done this, I was drinking much more water than usual and certainly a lot more than my team mates. I had a constant thirst and dry mouth. I could not stop eating, I needed to eat more and more and yet I never seemed to be full. Again, at first, I put this down to me being an active sportsman, I was literally playing sport all day at sixth form and then going training in the evenings, playing matches at weekends and having to do exercise and fitness sessions in between.

Eventually though, I realized my symptoms were beyond what would be considered normal. I now know all these symptoms are the classic symptoms of type one diabetes, but at the time I didn't know why I was feeling like this. When I now look back at the pictures from that match, I can see just how much weight I had lost and how ill I looked, but I still never thought I would have diabetes.

Fortunately, my Mum works in a local GP surgery in my home town and she knew that I was seriously ill. The Doctor arranged for me to go straight to the hospital ward where I was given a lot of tests, I specifically remember a lot of blood samples were taken. It all happened very quickly. It was then confirmed that I have Type 1 Diabetes, a condition I knew nothing about. What a steep learning curve the next few days, weeks and months would be!

I had to learn how to keep myself not only alive, but healthy. Initially, I was really surprised that I had Type 1 Diabetes, I knew nothing about it and I probably thought I couldn't get diabetes because I was young, fit and healthy. I imagined at first that I could cut things out of my diet or be prescribed some insulin and that was it. How wrong I was and if only it was that easy!

I remember the medical team at the hospital explaining everything to me; that it was just one of those things, it was not my fault, anyone can get it, there is no cure, I must test and inject every time I eat, this is not Type 2 Diabetes that we hear about on the news and so on. There was so much to take in, it was over whelming and I had so much to learn. This learning journey started by me throwing out any pre-conceived ideas I had about diabetes from the media and challenging any assumptions I had.

I had to learn how to test and interpret my blood sugars, learn what action to take and when, depending on the results. I had to learn how to test for ketones when my bloods are high or I feel unwell.

Injection techniques were demonstrated to me, I practiced a little bit, but really just had to get on with it and do it myself as I can no longer go more than a few hours without an injection. Carb counting was interesting, especially because I was on high carb diets due to the amount of sport I was playing at the time, I needed the extra energy and it soon got burnt off by me being active and I had to learn how to account for this when calculating insulin doses. I learned that without insulin, my body was not actually getting the energy from food, which was why I had been constantly hungry for the weeks leading up to my diagnosis. I also learned that my body was constantly dehydrated because my kidneys had been trying to flush the excess sugar from my body, so was using more water which then needed replacing. I learned how precious the human body is and how everything it needs has to be balanced out, having the right amount of the things that it needs at the right time. I guess you could say I had a newfound respect for my fitness and health, now I had to do a lot of extra work to look after myself.

Diabetes gives us so much to do, once I was well enough to leave hospital and the team were confident I knew what I was doing, I came home, but the team still kept coming to my house on home visits. My dietician came and taught me about the effects of different foods on the body, how they would affect me specifically and how I could still play sport. The dietician gave me lots of tips about how I could make carb counting more effective, fit into my lifestyle and also how to make carb counting and managing my diet easier now that I was living with diabetes. My Diabetes Specialist Nurse (**DSN**) also came to the house and we had a good talk about the day to day management, fitting diabetes into life rather than life into diabetes and she gave me some practical tips about management. Some of them were seemingly little things that are actually important, like how and when to order supplies on prescription, how to manage hypo's when out or even letting me know that I had free access to an **NHS Psychologist** if I felt I needed to talk to someone, or if I felt I was not coping.

Diabetes is a tough condition to manage, especially as I was 16, it was just a few weeks before my 17th birthday. My parents, family and friends were wonderfully supportive, but being diagnosed as an older teenager, I was expected to be in control of my care myself from day one. I already had a lot of freedom and my parents weren't with me all the time to keep an eye on me like they might be for a much younger child. I had to take control straight away, I think this is a good thing. I was diagnosed at an age where I had already spent time away from home without my parents, go away on lads' weekends, experimenting with alcohol, I was almost at driving age and I now had to do all this and look after my diabetes.

I'm sure anyone reading this book is aware that diabetes is a big cause of anxiety, there is so much to think about, our health is constantly on our minds. It was very overwhelming at first, even though I had amazing support from my family and the diabetes team, but I was very upset as I thought my cricket career had ended. Just keeping myself healthy now involved so much work, doing everyday activities like walking to school, crossing roads or having dinner late could actually be very dangerous if my numbers weren't in range. It seemed impossible that I could play sports at a professional level and also manage Type 1 Diabetes.

Playing Sport Again

It took me a long time to get used to living with Type 1, but I had to get used to it because living without it is not an option. I started to think about how I could manage this condition alongside playing professional sports that involve undertaking a high level of exercise and maintaining extreme fitness. My Doctors told me that if I managed it properly and had the commitment and dedication to both my health and my sport, there was no reason why I could not continue with my dream to play cricket at a professional level.

I was so pleased, I thought my health would get in the way of me achieving my lifelong dream, but I was wrong. I was certainly prepared to do anything I needed to do if it meant I could play professional cricket.

Looking back, I can see now that my diabetes actually helped to motivate me, both with playing cricket and having good control of my diabetes. I wasn't going to let my diagnosis stop me from playing my sport, so this motivated me to do whatever I needed to do to be able to play sport. If I am not healthy I cannot play, it is that simple just I now needed to work harder than my peers on maintaining my health. I had an extra thing I needed to do. It works both ways though, playing sport at professional level requires dedication and commitment for anyone and if I can apply this dedication and commitment to manage my condition then it will help me remain healthy. I can see how being a sportsman helps me with my diabetes care.

I went back to my sport, training and playing in matches. I have never been embarrassed by my diabetes, my friends in and outside of cricket are aware of my condition and have come to understand that sometimes I need time out to test, eat or treat a sneaky hypo. We are a tight knit community at Yorkshire Country Cricket Club (YCCC), so I just had to tell people there that I was now a person with diabetes and it wasn't a difficult or embarrassing thing to do. A lot of the lads were quite fascinated by it all and really took an interest. It took a while for them to understand and I don't think you can ever fully understand until you have lived with it, but they are great and a fantastic source of support to me. I do however remember one time my Jaffa cakes were stolen in the changing rooms, they very quickly learnt not to do that because I could need them in a true medical emergency. I took a light-hearted view to it, they didn't realise at that time just how serious it could have been. I guess it is all part of the camaraderie.

YCCC have been great, a lot of medical professionals are involved in professional sports anyway; such as dieticians advising us on nutrition, physio's helping us with injuries, medics and first aiders are there for accidents on the cricket field and we have to endure regular medical assessments and even massages! It was obvious to me that I needed to tell my coaches and the doctors at the cricket club about my diabetes so that they could best help and advise me, they are the professionals after all. I told them all about my treatments and what I need to stay healthy, they are then well informed as to how they can support me and help me play well for the team. My club have been wonderful, they look out for me and my diabetes has never been a problem. I don't see how it could be and I certainly wouldn't let it exclude me from anything.

I ended up working through the Yorkshire Cricket Academy, a program of intense training and sportsmanship. When I was 18 my childhood dream finally came true. I signed my first professional contract in the summer of 2018. I made my Twenty20 debut on 14th July, 2018 at the t20 blast in Worcester. I made my A list debut on 6th May, 2019, for Yorkshire in the 2019 Royal London One-Day Cup at Leeds. My first-class debut came the month after on 10th June, 2019, when I played for Yorkshire in the 2019 County Championship match at Guildford against Surrey.

I now get paid to play Cricket for Yorkshire at county level, this means playing in matches home and away, both in the UK and internationally. I get to spend a lot of time living in hotels! Managing diabetes when away is no different to when I am at home, it still involves the same amount of testing, I have to be organized with my supplies and monitor my diet.

Diabetes hasn't really impacted my career, but it does give me extra things to think about and manage. I am lucky that I have a lot of hypo awareness, so it is quite unusual for me to not spot a hypo. I can simply ask the staff to fetch my glucose if I feel a hypo coming on and this prevents any major medical disturbance to the cricket match. My team mates and the coaches are aware of how hypos could appear, they know the signs and symptoms so would always have this in the back of their minds if I ever was in a situation where I don't spot a hypo and they would remind me to test.

I have developed a very strict routine for my care, I have set times when I test. I test in the morning when I wake up, then again both before and after the warm up, then again just before we go onto the cricket field. If we are fielding I take some glucose tablets out on the field with me. I need to be really disciplined and keep on top of my routine in order to be successful. I have worked hard and have far too much to lose, I am not prepared to lose everything I have worked for.

Another example of how I keep to my strict routine is my diet. I will have the same breakfast every morning as I know how I respond to them. I can eat the breakfast and manage diabetes and I know exactly how my body responds and what my bloods will be two hours after testing. Being aware and knowing what will happen helps me predict and plan my day. Sometimes the cricket team are on tour and we will be playing away, this can involve having to eat different foods to those that my body is used to. Some hotels, especially the international ones, can serve bizarre things for breakfast! I try to stick to foods I am familiar with and I can predict what my bloods will be as far as it is possible to do so. If I do eat something different, I make sure I adjust my insulin, I might do an extra test and then I just get on with it.

It is also worth noting that I now test with a freestyle libre, so this makes it easier and is kinder on my fingers. I still inject though through my own choice, I inject my stomach. I wouldn't want a pump at the moment because I know that playing sports at this level will cause it to fall off or get hit and having to change a pump set during a match wouldn't be nice. I am happy with injections and I believe they actually make my life easier.

I have used my position to raise awareness of Type 1 Diabetes, the general public are not aware of what diabetes actually is and what living with it entails. I know I wasn't aware and I think that better awareness in society is needed. I am an ambassador for Diabetes UK, I put a Diabetes UK sticker on my bat for a year in order to raise awareness and to open up the conversations. Being an ambassador for Diabetes UK is a fantastic way for me to get involved with the diabetes community, raise awareness, get support and support others. I hope my experiences and my story will inspire other young people with diabetes, maybe they are struggling to cope and are worried about how the condition will affect their life, their hopes and dreams for the future. I believe diabetes doesn't have to stop you doing anything. Diabetes spurred me on, it was a big setback but one I wanted to overcome. I have earned a lot of respect from others by getting to the level I am at, despite living with diabetes.

Nothing is going to stop me now I am there, my next stop? Playing at country level and representing England!

My advice for people living with diabetes and their parents would be to develop your own routine, one that fits in to your life, don't let your life fit around diabetes, and then stick to it. You need to know when to test, when and what to eat, meal plan and don't rush the process as you are taking care of your health and that will pay dividends in the long run. Rushing through the process means mistakes can be made, invest time now into your health and the rewards will come.

Jordan's one tip for people with diabetes: develop a routine that works for you

Jordan's one tip for parents: support your child by helping them to implement their routine.

To see photo's of Jordan, check out our website at **www.typeawesome.co.uk**

Chapter 6

'Travelling through life with Type 1 Diabetes."

Lydia Parkhurst

Lydia was diagnosed when she was 12 years old, just after a family holiday abroad. All Lydia ever wanted to do was to travel the world and study Geography at University. Lydia was determined to not let it prevent her from discovering the world and exploring other cultures. Lydia is very active in the Type 1 Community, relentlessly campaigning for change and having met Theresa May and Ed Milliband. She documents her travels on her blog "The Backpacker and the Pod", which inspires others with diabetes to travel and gives tips on the practicalities of doing so. Lydia achieved her other aim of passing her Geography degree, where she specialized in Health Geography, completing her dissertation on the inequalities in healthcare.

Lydia now teaches Geography in her home town of Doncaster, South Yorkshire, but gets itchy feet and pre-covid, would often be seen with a camera and a flight
ticket in her hand, about to jet off somewhere to photograph her adventures. Lydia tells us about her first independent travelling, where she inter-railed around Europe with some friends.

Summer 2017, I was to set off on the biggest adventure of my life at that point, I was planning an inter-railing trip around Europe with two of my best friends, Alice and Sophie. We had planned for months, looking at different locations and laughing at the names of the dodgy hostels we would be staying in, *ahem* *'my sweet home forever'* to name one! We would be staying in plenty of hostels, travelling on trains and visiting 7 different countries throughout the trip.

Many teenagers go on adventures like this, but this trip involved a lot more planning for me because 7 years before, when I was 12, I was diagnosed with Type 1 Diabetes. At the time of my trip, I wore an Omnipod tubeless pump to deliver insulin and a Libre flash glucose monitor. This trip was to be my first time travelling abroad with this bionic equipment, previous overseas adventures had involved finger pricking and injecting.

The route

Warsaw - Poland

Auschwitz - Poland

Salzburg - Austria

Innsbruck - Austria

Lake Bled - Slovenia

Venice - Italy

Pisa - Italy

Rome - Italy

Tirano - Italy/Switzerland

Chur - Switzerland

Lucerne - Switzerland

Montreux - Switzerland

Paris - France

Amsterdam - Netherlands

The adventure was so exciting and T1D did not stop me exploring! I will tell you about my trip whilst also giving some of my top tips for backpacking and inter-railing abroad when living with Type 1 Diabetes.

Medicine, medicine everywhere... But what if I run out?

We have two rules in my house which I considered when packing. Write down all your carb ratio's, background insulin, hourly basal rates for every hour of the day and emergency telephone numbers; and **times by two, divide and spare**. Sounds like a math's equation, so let me explain ...

1. **TIMES BY TWO** - Take twice as much insulin and supplies than you would normally need! If you normally have 5 tests a day, plan for 10, take double the number of pods, pump supplies, insulin pens, vials etc. It is always better to have it with you. In this case however I took a cannula for each day - purely because I knew from prior experience that sun cream is brilliant at unsticking cannulas and I'm very clumsy at walking into door frames and ripping my cannula from my arm!

2. **DIVIDE** - Split the medicine and supplies into different bags (and always in hand luggage!) This stops it getting lost when the hold bag goes missing and it has less chance of getting broken! I was extremely lucky that my two friends were so supportive and helped carry my medicine around Europe for me. I therefore was able to have cannulas in each of their hand luggage along with a spare blood sugar handset and Frio pack with 2 bottles of insulin. It is also worth noting that goods in the hold of a plane can freeze, frozen insulin is no good! NEVER put any insulin in the hold of a plane.

3. **SPARE** - Along with my 10 cannulas and my Frio pack with my insulin vials for my pump and everything else that goes with my Omnipod; (strips, batteries, glucose tablets and lancets,) I brought spare handsets; a blood glucose handset, a ketone machine and a spare handset which Omnipod kindly loaned me through their holiday PDM service - LIFESAVER if something was to go wrong! Insulin pens and needles were also packed in case the Omnipod got thrown off a cliff or sunk to the bottom of a lake! Thankfully I didn't have to use any of these but if they weren't packed... they would have been needed!

BUT WHAT IF I RUN OUT?! - Along with my passport, diabetes letters for the airport and details of my route I wrote down the supply numbers for each country I was going too, so I could ring

them if I needed any emergency supplies, however, if it is just test strips, batteries or your blood glucose monitor that has broken, you can buy these from the nearest pharmacy.

Bum-bags are the best thing to carry your day medicine in. Handy and less likely to get pick pocketed than your rucksack! I only took out the spares I may have needed for that day. Just make sure than you lock the rest in a locker in the hostel.

Always be prepared for airport security!

Along with the holiday PDM, I asked my language teachers to translate a document for me to explain that it if go through an airport scanner with my handset and pod, they could break. This was really useful to have in addition to my GP and Diabetes Specialist Nurse letters. I took my translated letter with me to any attractions I visited in case they used scanners and it made my life so much easier than trying to play charades or say 'like pacemaker' which actually usually does the trick!

I had a really positive experience at the airport in the UK on our flight out and at Amsterdam airport on our flight home. It is really fantastic how far technology and awareness has come. At the time I went travelling, the security at Amsterdam had never seen an Omnipod. There are always so many opportunities to educate people about Type 1 Diabetes!

Insurance

Insure your pump! My Omnipod was insured through our household insurance but it wasn't cheap! Not only did we have to insure my handset but also each pod which I took away! EEEK! On top of equipment insurance, I needed insurance for me! We insured through 'Essential Travel' for backpackers and it only cost £50 which was really good. I have since used them again for future adventures!

Alarms and testing

Alarms were my lifesaver during Inter-railing. Although after arriving in Poland I didn't have to change the time zones on my

pump as all the countries we visited were all one hour ahead, when you are busy you still forget to test. Every day, my alarms on my phone would chime to remind me to test, this happened at 7:30 am when we woke up, 10am, 12pm lunchtime, 2pm, 5pm dinnertime and 9pm (close to bedtime some nights!). Although sometimes it wasn't convenient to test, such as on the busy metro in France, it helped me keep a closer eye on my bloods which was needed in such varying environments!

FOOD

Always take spare food! I took a few boxes of cereal bars for emergencies. When we arrived in Oświęscim (the town of Auschwitz) it was late and it was very difficult to buy food! Thankfully we found a Tesco supermarket in the quiet town, it was just about to shut so we ran in to grab some food!

Heat and diabetes... and the fact that every time you see a famous landmark you go low.

Heat affects everybody's diabetes differently. I know lots of my friends go low in the heat, but I go high. All the more reason for extra tests, I know it is a cliché and the last thing you want to do, but it is the only way you can properly manage and prevent major incidents. Walking makes me go low, as I already knew from doing my Duke of Edinburgh awards. So, with walking and the heat, I had no idea what was going to happen to my bloods but I hoped they would be balanced in the middle of high and low. Walking combatted the heat and I was low more than I was high. Thank goodness I packed so many glucotabs! However, I didn't use any temporary basal rates as the low was only once a day and at an unpredictable time. It was a little bit annoying though when you don't really get to appreciate the Leaning Tower of Pisa as you guzzle Sprite and trying not to get pick pocketed!

Diet coke and coke zero?!?

Be prepared to spend more than your friend drinking full sugar drinks because nearly everywhere charged more for diet coke. Also, most European countries, excluding Italy, seem to have something against Diet Coke. They only have Coke Zero, which by the way, does not taste the same.

Seeing double?

I was walking around Lucerne with my Libre on the back of one arm and my Omnipod on the back of my other arm, admiring my surroundings when a teenage boy, a similar age to myself, tapped me on my libre. I turned around to see him holding a Libre handset. I panicked thinking I had dropped my handset, frantically feeling in my bum-bag. I pulled out my Libre handset. All of a sudden, I was seeing double. He was Type 1 as well and he was trying to show me his Libre! Despite the language barrier we chatted about the Libre and took a photo! It's not often you meet other people who live with Type 1 Diabetes!

Fragile feet

Oh, my goodness! Don't get me started talking about my poor feet! By the time we arrived in Lucerne (17 days into our trip) my feet were very sore! Much to the despair of my parents, I did not take walking shoes! I took my running trainers which I wear at home, however as we were averaging 10 miles a day and it was hot, I developed blisters. I had blisters on both little toes (which was expected) and a gigantic blister on my right ball of my foot. The blister popped and my raw foot was agony. *TOP TIP* Always listen to your mum and dad! After using some Mepore dressing and taking some antibiotics, it started to heal. Until it turns out I'm allergic to Penicillin! I have now found out that if you smother your feet in Vaseline before putting your socks and shoes on you don't get the friction so you don't get the blisters!

People abroad use your diabetes as a chat up line!

Oh my gosh! Never in my life have so many people asked me about my insulin pump, and adding to that, known the difference between Type 1 and Type 2 without having to be told. I was gob smacked! Especially when people go out of the way to talk to you about it, like the time we were sitting having a pizza in Innsbruck, Austria, and a man on the table next to us turned around and asked me what the thing was on my arm (my pump), he already knew about type 1 and 2 and was lovely to talk too. Normally people stare and mutter to their friend that it is a nicotine patch and its terrible that I smoked! (Which I don't).

The second occasion was in Lake Bled, Slovenia, at our Hostel '*Ace of Spades*'. Whilst booking in the man asked me what was on my arm, and again I explained. It turned out one of his family members had type 1, and this conversation led to the lady who worked there telling me she was a dietician! I would definitely recommend visiting Lake Bled. THE most beautiful place on our trip!

However, in Salzburg, at the youth hostel, the barman, instead of the generic questions about my pump, used my diabetes as a chat up

line! The barman already knew about Type 1 diabetes and insulin pumps and he went out of his way to find me the last diet coke! He then came and sat with us over dinner and asked if he could prick my finger. Such a funny and nice guy who I have to say, is the first person to chat me up with my diabetes!

AND FINALLY HAVE FUN!

Don't let diabetes get in the way of you doing anything! Yes, testing more is inconvenient and so is hypoing in the middle of the metro carrying a 65-litre rucksack and a daypack, but you can do it! I did it! Yes, it's a challenge but at the end of the day you only live life at the end of your comfort zone and we can do anything anyone else can do – just with Type 1 Diabetes! I would definitely recommend getting a medical alert bracelet for travelling as it put my mind so much more at ease knowing that if I had a problem someone would have a better idea why. It was such an amazing experience and I hope that what I've learnt will help you too!

Other adventures
Diabetes has given me the opportunity to raise awareness on an international level and to meet some incredible people.
I have had the amazing opportunity to meet Theresa May (who also has Type 1) when she was the serving Prime Minister, Leader of the Opposition at the time Rt. Hon Ed Miliband and I have met HRH The Duchess of Cornwall.

Meeting a Duchess and a Prime Minister

I was invited to The Guildhall in London by JDRF, when I arrived, I was told I would be speaking to the then Prime Minister Theresa May. Fair to say I was very nervous!
However, after shaking her hand and being told to address her informally as Theresa, my nerves disappeared. We chatted about our diagnosis's, and how Theresa managed her diabetes through her hectic schedule. We also spoke about my blog and how raising awareness for Type 1 was so important. I showed Theresa that I wore my insulin pump on one arm and my Freestyle Libre on the other and that I didn't mind wearing my devices so publicly because it raises awareness. Theresa told me that she was just about to start using the Libre, so I couldn't help giving her a tip! It was such a fantastic experience being able to talk to such a lovely and influential person about a disease we both face day in and day out. I also found out Theresa did a geography degree. We already have two similarities! - Does this mean I could be Prime Minister in the future?! Speaking to Theresa's PA afterwards she said she was impressed with how articulate I was when speaking to Theresa, I think I left an impression - and we were asked down to Downing Street for a private tour!

One other person I met on this trip was a man who has lived with Type 1 diabetes for 70 years. When I was talking to him, he told me that he was on injections and that he uses a Dexcom. Pulling the Dexcom receiver out of his pocket he had the straightest line of around 6.5mmol! He told me he had no complications as a result of his Type 1 and he had no complication with his eyes. This man is my new inspiration. This just shows that you can do anything with Type 1 and live a normal and healthy life.

Throughout the evening I spoke to many parents and JDRF supporters about my Omnipod, which I was wearing on the back of my arm. By the end of the evening my Pod was referred to as the 'party pod' because it was painted with nail varnish. My pod also caught the attention of HRH The Duchess of Cornwall's Personal Assistant. I was invited to speak to HRH The Duchess of Cornwall about my insulin pump and I explained to the Duchess that I always wear my pump with pride because I make 100's of important decisions every day to manage my diabetes. I was asked by The Duchess if lots of people ask what my Pod was. Laughing and chatting I told The Duchess that I used to tell the Beaver Scouts that I was part robot as it was hard to explain to young children, cue laughter from everyone around us! It was such a nerve racking and amazing experience speaking to The Duchess and my blood sugars completely agreed with the adrenaline I was feeling! Straight line on my libre going up!

Visiting 10 Downing Street

When you get diagnosed with Type 1 you're often told that the condition doesn't stop you doing anything (apart from being in the army or being an astronaut) but sometimes it's hard to actually believe this, especially when the person telling you this doesn't often live with diabetes.

However, standing at 10 Downing Street, I felt a sense of pride. Whether you support the Conservative Party, the Labour Party or any other, Theresa May shows us that type 1 diabetes has not held her back.

For me this shows her as a positive role model, showing all of us that we can do whatever we want and although diabetes may make it a little trickier, or we have to take a different path, we can achieve our dreams.

I have been incredibly lucky to travel around the world telling my story of my life with Type 1, travelling to South Korea to speak at one of the largest diabetes conferences in the world. I have participated in round tables for companies such as the Guardian, to raise awareness and support for Young Peoples Transition Services. I was sponsored by Abbott to attend the diabetes bloggers programme at #DXStockholm. I enjoy volunteering at local Diabetes Camps, helping younger people to take control of their Type 1, I think it really helps them to learn from others who have type1 themselves.

My top tip - Don't be afraid to chase your dreams. My parents, sister and family have always been a massive part of helping me achieve mine - they have believed in me and helped me from day one. I feel so lucky that I have such a supportive family and as a family we live by the motto that diabetes doesn't stop you achieving anything you put your mind to. Sometimes, it just requires a little more planning. Every dream starts with a plan and an "I can."

Lydia has a blog, "The Backpacker and the Pod" where she documents her travels, public speaking, events & adventures with T1D:

https://thebackpackerandthepod.wordpress.com/

To keep up to date with Lydia and to see photo's of her adventures, check out our website at **www.typeawesome.co.uk**

Chapter 7

"I can now soar through my day without the fear that diabetes will stop me"

Laura Dunion

Laura is a young lady who is truly inspirational, so inspirational in fact that she now has letters after her name after receiving a British Citizen Award in 2020 for her services in volunteering and charitable giving. Laura's campaigns include raising awareness of Type 1 Diabetes, fundraising over £90,000, public speaking, her role in the Artificial Pancreas clinical trial in 2014 and then subsequently being one of the first people in the UK to use the Medtronic MiniMed 670G insulin pump, a revolutionary technology that uses a hybrid closed loop system to manage Type 1 Diabetes. Now widely available, this device has changed the lives of many people with T1D.

Laura was diagnosed aged 8 and is now 19 years old and a student at Leeds Beckett University, where she is studying Youth Work and Community
Development. Laura has not let diabetes get in the way of her life, she has always embraced the condition and used it to bring about change. Laura's work has taken her to UK Parliament and also Capitol Hill in Washington DC, America, where she was chosen to represent the UK at JDRF Children's Congress. Oh yes, she has also climbed Mont Blanc. Let's learn more about this incredible and selfless young lady.

I was 8 years old, almost 9, I had just started getting a little bit of independence as this was the age my Mum had just started letting me play out on the street with some friends without her having to watch me all the time and trusting me to walk to a friend's house nearby on my own. This all changed when I was diagnosed with Type One Diabetes.

When I was 8, this independence was threatened when I became ill. The typical symptoms of Type One are known as "the 4 T's" - thirst, toilet, thinner, tired. Patients usually experience insatiable thirst, increase in toilet visits and excess urination, they lose weight so become thinner - the weight loss can be excessive and lastly, extreme tiredness occurs as the body has no energy from glucose because insulin is not present in the body to move it to the appropriate places. Other symptoms can also be present, like general malaise, headaches, dry skin and blurry vision, but the four T's are the classic ones to look out for. Luckily for me, my Mum was aware of the symptoms of Type One and had identified them in me, so I went to the GP and was diagnosed. It was 15th February 2010, I do not remember much at all about my diagnosis, but my Mum does and she has recalled it as below:

I took Laura to our GP as she had been drinking lots and was very tired. It was an evening appointment at about 6:30pm. In the back of my mind I had thought
about Type 1 Diabetes however I had ruled this thought out quickly and blamed it on a urine infection. We took a urine sample with us and our GP tested it and looked shocked at the result. The Glucose reading was very high. She then used a blood monitor and did a finger prick test. This only showed a slight increase in glucose above a normal level however our GP had found it difficult to get the monitor to work initially.
She contacted the hospital and they advised for us to go home and go down to the hospital in the morning.
An hour later there was a knock at my front door and when I answered it I found our GP standing there looking worried. She explained that we may think she was slightly mad, however she said she wouldn't sleep tonight if she didn't check

Laura's BG again. The urine test result had been so different to the BG result she was concerned that the original monitor wasn't working properly. She tested Laura's BG again and it just read HI. She contacted the hospital and we had to
go there immediately. What a fantastic GP. I will never forget her and I told her this once a couple of years later when I saw her again and thanked her for being so
vigilant. She also said that she would never forget us and told us that GPs may only ever diagnose one child with Type 1 in their whole careers and we were her one.

Importance of diagnosis

Sometimes, the symptoms are missed or are hidden due to another illness, sadly undiagnosed Type 1 always leads to coma and coma often leads to fatalities. It is therefore really important to get medical help immediately if you or anyone you know has any of these symptoms, a quick dip of the urine or a quick finger prick blood test, is all it initially takes to test for high levels of sugar in the body. This is also why paramedics and A&E departments finger prick test all patients, even if they have seemingly unrelated symptoms, because as I stated, the signs of T1 can be hidden so only the signs of infection would show.

My Diagnosis

I was too young to understand everything that was going on, but I can remember that there was a big fuss and my diagnosis shocked everyone, not least my parents who were beside themselves with worry. Whilst in hospital, I met my fabulous consultant Dr Fiona Campbell. I met Fiona, my amazing nurse Jane and the fantastic team at Leeds Children's Hospital in my first week after diagnosis. I spent 6 days in hospital learning how to Carb count, test and inject. I was on Multiple Daily Injections (MDI) when I left. Before I left we had a conversation about insulin pumps. They asked me if I would like one as it would mean I would do less injections and it would be a bit easier. They showed me some brochures about pumps, one of them came in pink. The decision was made!

It was a very steep learning curve for me and everyone who took care of me and spent time with me - my parents, my brother, extended family & friends, teachers, after school clubs and my dance teacher. We had no other option but to learn and just get on with it. My Mum has since said she felt like she was starting again as a parent as it is like having a new-born baby, she had a new set of rules now and had to watch me all the time, she couldn't let me out of her sight in fear I would have a hypo. Just like having a new-born, Mum also had to get up through the night to test and correct my blood sugars, but even on the nights they were relatively stable, she wouldn't sleep because she knew the situation could have changed at any point and without notice, as I could have gone too low or too high without warning; that's what type 1 diabetes does! Mum couldn't even leave me alone in another room of the house without worrying because at any point I could have collapsed from low blood sugars.

Over time, life did get easier and Mum learnt how to look after me, help me look after myself and also how to start letting go and have the independence my peers had. I am sure it was incredibly hard for her, but as a family, we had support from an excellent charity called Juvenile Diabetes Research Foundation (JDRF). I believe our involvement with JDRF dramatically changed our lives for the better and allowed us to feel more in control of this diabetes monster. JDRF organize "Discovery Days" where we would not only meet other families going through the same as us, but also be educated on current trials and treatments that can potentially improve management of, or even cure diabetes. Going to these events we felt less isolated, more supported, more in control of our future and we had increased hope for a cure, we even sometimes got to meet the scientists who are developing the potential cures! I made many friends my own age who also had Type 1 Diabetes, I would sometimes see these in clinic or on camp too and we would support each other. It is different to be with someone who actually knows

what diabetes feels like. JDRF have been very helpful to me and my family and I am very grateful for all the work that they do.

Volunteering

I have volunteered with several diabetes charities over the last few years, I believe it is important to give back. It is also a great way to meet others, get support, share stories and keep up to date with developments.

I have volunteered with JDRF as a way of giving back for the support I have received from them, I even became a JDRF Youth Ambassador. I have helped in many ways; I have presented at Discovery Days, helped at fun runs selling T-Shirts and even at one event I was responsible for setting up and running the bouncy castle!

I visited Anfield Stadium, the home of Liverpool Football Club, for a Discovery Day and I got to see the incredible amount of work and effort that goes into organizing and delivering an event and then seeing the families arrive. The JDRF staff are very welcoming, friendly and supportive and I am proud to work alongside them. A lot of the events are far away from my home in Leeds, so I often have to get up very early but I really don't mind as I know I will be helping other families in a similar way that JDRF helped my family after diagnosis. Mum says she has never seen me so motivated as she does on those early mornings I am volunteering for JDRF.

At the events, people ask me a lot of questions about my diabetes, my insulin pump and continuous glucose monitor (CGM), I really enjoy showing other people the technology available, giving them the positive information about the equipment and answering any questions they may have. I also try to inspire them and help them see that Type 1 Diabetes doesn't have to stop you from doing anything. I especially enjoy interacting with the children and I try to be a positive role model for them, many of them have not met a person with Type 1 prior to coming to the event. Sometimes, I even get to look after small groups of children with diabetes whilst their parents go off to listen to the talks. I really enjoy doing this as I know I am helping the whole family.

I have often spoken about my volunteering role in other areas of life, such as giving talks at school assemblies, when at my own diabetes appointments and even at my college interview.
Volunteering has helped me to manage my own condition, improve understanding and even get on my college and university course. I especially found that the work experience element of volunteering has helped me in my chosen field of work.

I was lucky to gain some work experience at Leeds Children's Hospital where I shadowed play therapists, I am certain that my experiences with JDRF helped me to secure this. I also became a member of the Leeds Hospital Youth Forum where I work alongside children with a wide range of chronic health conditions to advocate for our rights, ensure our voices can be heard and to campaign to improve facilities & resources at the hospital. I also became involved with the fantastic organization DigiBete. DigiBete are a not for profit organization set up by the parents of a child with Type 1, they work in partnership with the Diabetes Team at Leeds Children's Hospital to bring medically accurate resources to help children, young people and their families self-manage Type One Diabetes. DigiBete have a full clinically approved training platform to raise awareness, and provide support, education & training about Type 1 Diabetes. I have taken part in filming some of their resources, which give other young people and their families a greater, more practical insight into living with Type 1. I also support young people and children at local DigiBete social events and I am now an ambassador for this organization too.

Artificial Pancreas and Medtronic Minimed 670G Pump

My involvement with my own diabetes care led to an amazing opportunity in 2014 when I was asked by my Diabetes Team in Leeds to take part in a pioneering Artificial Pancreas clinical trial. I was one of the first children in the world to trial this system outside of a hospital environment. The Artificial Pancreas used an insulin pump, continuous glucose monitor and a complex algorithm. I used the Artificial Pancreas every night for three months, it constantly monitored my blood glucose levels and adjusted the insulin that was required, keeping my blood glucose in perfect range night after night. It meant my Mum did not have to check me throughout the night and for the first time in 4 years, she could sleep knowing that I was safe and that I would not go low, which can be life-threatening, or have long term complications linked to high blood glucose levels. The biggest fear for my Mum has always been me going low in the night. I think this is the same for all parents of Type 1 children and young people.

The technology gave us hope, freedom and reduced anxieties. It was very difficult to hand it back, after the trial, as we had got so used to it over the trial period. When we did hand it back, we knew that we had been part of a revolutionary development in Type 1 diabetes management that would help thousands of people all over the world.

Following the trial, I started on the Medtronic Minimed 640G which was similar in that it could suspend insulin when a low blood glucose level was predicted, however, it couldn't deliver any additional insulin if blood glucose levels went high. The Artificial Pancreas trial was funded by JDRF and was an overwhelming success and this led to other systems being developed.

I was absolutely delighted in November 2018 when I was one of the first people in the UK to get the amazing Medtronic MiniMed 670G. The Medtronic Minimed 670G is the first insulin pump that uses new technology known as a hybrid closed loop system. It can detect patterns of blood glucose levels and suspend insulin delivery when blood glucose goes low and increase insulin delivery when blood glucose goes high. Just like the technology used in the Artificial Pancreas trial, it works using an insulin pump, a complex algorithm and a continuous glucose monitor. The insulin is delivered via an infusion set which I wear on my stomach. The Medtronic Minimed 670G aims to keep my blood glucose in a safe level 24 hours a day. It is not fully automatic, for example, it does not work quick enough when eating so I still have to manually tell it how many carbohydrates I have eaten and it then works out how much insulin to deliver. It has been revolutionary in the management of my Type 1 Diabetes and certainly feels like a cure! I was involved in lots of media work when I got the 670G including being on the front page of our local newspaper with my amazing consultant Dr Fiona Campbell and doing a media story for BBC news which was shown on news bulletins throughout the day. The story was also featured in several newspapers all over the country. It was fantastic and raised lots of awareness about Type 1 Diabetes and the importance of Technology to help manage it. I have since then spoken about this Technology at several JDRF Discovery Days and for the very powerful and emotive JDRF Lifeline appeal which was featured on the BBC in July 2019.

The Medtronic MiniMed 670G is widely available whenever it is clinically necessary and Medtronic have just launched an even more advanced model of this system called the Medtronic Minimed 780G which I should be transferring on to in November 2020. This system is described as an Advanced Hybrid Closed Loop and will have even more amazing features than the 670G. I am so excited to be able to access this technology and I will be helping my clinic again by providing lots of feedback about this system and continuing to report about my Type 1 Tech journey.

The 670G has given me a huge amount of freedom, I can now soar through my day without the fear that diabetes will stop me. I have always tried hard to never let Diabetes stop me doing anything, however, if I was doing something and had a hypo, I would have to stop until I had tested, treated, re-tested and felt OK. I rarely have highs and lows now, certainly not to the extremes I did pre-the 670G. It has even given me the confidence to learn to drive and live independently at university without worrying about a hypo spoiling things or endangering my life, or in the case of driving, endangering the lives of other people.

It also came at a good time in my life, it meant my Mum was more relaxed about me going out, drinking, going to university, going on holidays with my friends and I guess eventually leaving home. Most importantly it has reassured her that I will be safe overnight and not at risk of going hypo in my sleep.

America

One of my greatest achievements so far was being selected to represent the UK at JDRF's Children's Congress in Washington DC in the summer of 2017. My volunteering experience definitely played a huge part in me being selected to take part in this incredible opportunity. I was delighted and felt honoured to be participating in this event and to be a voice for children in the UK who live with type 1 diabetes. My role, along with 150 other children with T1 from around America and the world, was to visit Capitol Hill,

to convince US Federal Lawmakers, to continue funding JDRF to find a cure. The American Government gives $150 million a year to JDRF and the Children's Congress works hard to make sure this funding keeps coming in. I met Congressmen and Senators in America's corridors of power. I had only ever seen these people and buildings on TV, but here I was not only physically there, but making a difference influencing them as to where America's money is best spent. I took part in radio and TV interviews as well as a big social media campaign. We were successful at securing the funding and now, because of my trip, $150 million a year continues to fund much needed research into potential cures for Type One Diabetes. After seeing and experiencing myself just how far research and treatments have advanced in the 10 years since my diagnosis, I am confident that JDRF will achieve their aim to find a cure for this condition.

Mont Blanc

Another big personal challenge I undertook was taking part in the T1D Challenge -Tour de Mount Blanc, supported by the Sweet Project, World Diabetes Tour and Sanofi. Along with 9 other young people who live with T1 from around the world, I was invited to "Tour de Mont Blanc" - a week long trek around the Mont Blanc mountain range, trekking 20 km a day and venturing into Switzerland, Italy and France. France had the imposing glaziers, Italy had giant granite rock faces and Switzerland had the long, smooth valleys. This trek sure was a challenge, type 1 or not!

At first, we did wonder if I can undertake this incredible challenge, not just because of the physical and medical side, but the fact I would have no access to make up, hairdryers or straighteners for a whole week! I looked at previous videos of the expedition and all the literature about the route and it made me even more motivated to do it, even though I couldn't take my make up! I learned that I would be supported by Doctors, mentors, dieticians and other health care professionals who either had Type 1 themselves or were experts in this field, some were both.

It took a lot of planning. We had meetings with my team, including an in-depth meeting with my fantastic Dietician Frances Hansen, to discuss the amount of carbs that I would potentially need on the trip. I would be carrying everything, including hypo treatments, snacks, clothes and T1 supplies. The bag was packed and repacked several times to squeeze everything in. I had to do lots of taste testing and label checking to make sure snacks contained the highest amount of carbs we could find - with the lightest weight.

Then came the training. I had never done any trekking before; however, I was physically fit and just needed to improve my stamina and strength. I only had a couple of months until the Trek and I was busy at college so I had to fit in the training around an already busy schedule. I had some sessions with a personal trainer who was also my Biology Tutor so that helped, and I did some cycling with my Dad and on a cycling machine at home. The dog also got a lot of walks around this time!

Finally, the big day came and I was all packed up and ready to go. I did not have any worries or fears about doing the Trek., I couldn't wait to go. My Mum on the other hand was a nervous wreck! I flew to Geneva, where I met one of the consultants called Olga and one of the young people called Pia who were both from Germany. I said my goodbyes to my parents who kindly flew over with me as it would have been the first time in another country without them.

The taxi ride was a bit awkward as I didn't know the consultant or Pia plus they knew each other and were talking in German so I had no idea what they were saying. When we arrived at the hotel it turned out me and Pia were going to be roommates that night. Pia was very good at speaking English and we soon became good friends.

That night we had to put on Dexcom's which we had to wear to provide data about our blood glucose levels and we also made a video of what we wanted to get out of the trek. This was funny as we all had no idea what was going on but it helped as it meant we had time to socialise and get to know each other better.
The morning after it was time to start the Trek.
 Honestly it felt like I was not prepared at all. I can't remember much of the first day as the week just blended into one.

So, I'll just tell you about my highlights of the week.

- On one of the days we had to slide on our bags down some snow which was really fun.
- On another we came to a stop for a picture but the camera man was taking his time to get ready so it turned into a big snow ball fight.
- Every time we stopped for lunch we had amazing views. Sometimes we stopped at a lake, one time we stopped in a hut where it was so dark we had to use our head torches.
- We trekked through sun, rain, winds, and hail storms.
- Pia, Thibo from Belgium, Efe from Turkey and I were all walking down together and decided to put on some music and we all started signing our hearts out. This was one of my favourite memories.
- We had to walk across some serious bridges which did not feel safe at all.
- We stayed in refuges which were alright, but one night I had to wash my hair in a sink as all the showers didn't last long.
- Another time the showers were freezing cold and we were all screaming in them.
- At night all the young people shared a room. #noprivacy.
- Imagine one large bunk bed with 10 mattresses on top and 10 below all alongside each other and with me being the smallest I got to sleep on the smallest mattress.
- Every night someone's CGM alarm would be going off. One-time Efe's blood went low and he kept shouting that he needed to eat but he didn't want to eat. We were all laughing at him as we understood how he was feeling and we all stayed up to make sure he ate and was ok.
- Another time we had a shush competition as everyone used to shush when alarms went off.
- Every day I would be the last one at the top of the mountain but the first at the bottom. I struggled walking up but walking down was easy.

- One day we had a choice of going to the shops or going to the refuge – to get first choice for the beds. I chose to go to the refuge. I like my bed!!
- When the others got back Mike Riddell – one of the mentors brought me back some lovely crisps which made my day.
- My Blood levels were up and down just like the mountains. Every day was different and it was hard to know what to change on my insulin settings. I decreased my insulin as the days went on from 75% then to 50%. I was always supported by the Doctors.
- On one day I had a 1.8 which I have never had before. I was fine though and just sat and looked at the views. It was quite a nice place to have a hypo.
- I had to eat lots of my carby snacks just to keep my blood sugar up.

Despite all of the challenges the Trek was one of the best experiences in my life so far. The friends I made will be friends for life. It was absolutely fantastic. It boosted my confidence to be more independent and I loved it.

British Citizen Award

In January 2020, I went to The Palace of Westminster in London to receive a British Citizen Award for Volunteering and Charitable giving. The medal presentation was hosted at the House of Lords by television presenter Michael Underwood, who along with Dame Mary Perkins, is a patron of the British Citizen Award. It was an honour to be recognized for the work that I do, it is work I hope to be involved with for a long time to come.

I continue to share my story and help others and I have even been able to do this recently by participating in a JDRF Virtual Discovery Day.

Type 1 Diabetes is my friend and not my enemy. It has helped me grow and develop as a person and it is part of who I am. I want to use all of the fantastic opportunities that I have been given to inspire other young people and show them that Type 1 Diabetes should not stop them from doing what they want to do. I am now in my second year at university pursing my goal in life to be a Hospital Youth Worker and I am living life to the full.

Digibete, who Laura volunteers with, are an organization who have a video platform to share videos and educational resources about Type 1 Diabetes. The content is designed to help support children, young people and families to self manage their own diabetes by extending the reach of clinical teams online. Digibete's mission is to increase education, awareness and training for Type 1 Diabetes.

Digibete can be found at:
www.digibete.org

To find out more about Laura and to see photo's of her amazing achievements, check out the website at **www.typeawesome.co.uk**

Chapter 8

"50 years living with Type 1 Diabetes"

Mary Hayes

Mary has lived a fulfilling life despite having lived with Type 1 Diabetes since she was 10 years old. Mary worked hard and gained her nursing degree, a master's degree and then used her experience to help others living with diabetes so became a Diabetes Specialist Nurse (DSN) herself. Mary has used her skills in the UK but has also given international talks at diabetes conferences, in addition to becoming the first person from overseas to visit Dr Pendsey in India. Mary enjoys spending time with her husband, children and grandchildren, but found it hard to retire so now continues her nursing work part time, alongside supporting The Pendsey Trust.

Living with type 1 diabetes is not a normal life, whatever that might be, but to me it is still a life worth living. Over the years I have learnt to live with it, just like you would learn to live with an old family relative; most of the time it is a familiar friend and feels comfortable, but then it can be really frustrating when you least expect it.
It is the most annoying thing in the world and I feel there is nothing much you can do about it, other than just get on with it and enjoy your life!

It was May 1971, I was ten years old. I had lost a lot of weight so my mother had tried feeding me extra cake, she made me go to the farm yard every week to be weighed on the potato scales as they were regularly checked for accuracy. Weight loss was the main symptom, Mother realised I wasn't well when the weight just kept falling off. Mother took me to the GP and told she recalled a child she had taught who had diabetes, to which my Mother was told by the GP that she was "an over anxious housewife and should get a hobby". She persisted with a urine sample which when tested turned orange. Calmly, he said I should be tested as a precaution and he wrote to the hospital. In the meantime, I should avoid carbohydrates. I disliked the school potatoes and puddings so was delighted to announce I cannot have this as I am a diabetic. The look on the dinner ladies face when she put the spoon down, she looked grave and went into the kitchen to tell the others. I can remember it now as clear as day, her face and her actions told me that a child living with this is not good. In hindsight, I can see how maybe she was upset by this news.

I remember the day I had a full glucose tolerance test. We received a results letter in the post asking us to attend an outpatient appointment. At this appointment I was diagnosed with Type 1 Diabetes and rushed into hospital!

I cried when I went into hospital, I was brought up on a farm with my brother and sister, we had holidayed every year but I had never really been away from my family and I certainly had no experience of hospitals. I cried because I was left alone there, I can remember the ward sister telling me not to cry because I was upsetting my mother. The hospital was now my home for two weeks while
I learned how to manage my newly diagnosed Type 1 Diabetes. In those days, they didn't talk to the patient as such, I was never told I would have diabetes and need to inject for the rest of my life. I loved the nurses, the hospital Sunday school and the school classes. I spent ages trying not to do my first injection, I remember pretending that it

wouldn't go in. The nurse suggested that if I didn't hurry up I would miss breakfast, I could see the other children at the trolley which ended up being my cue to just get on with it. Mother learnt to inject me but my Father would not, the ward Sister said I could not go home until he had. Mother explained I would have to stay in hospital then, because he did not inject his pigs so he wouldn't be injecting his precious daughter. I made a little note of that and was horrified when I went home the next day as my mother had won her battle. I thought I would be staying, my little holiday was over! Dad never injected me but he played his part and took me to all my hospital appointments and learnt to inject his pigs.

Every day, as she drew up my insulin Mother said, "God bless Banting and Best". She was a firm mother and she did not really 'do' illness. Anything medical she was faintly and gave my insulin too shallow leaving a lump. After one such occasion I asked her to let me give my insulin as I had in hospital and she agreed. Before long she started saying "Mary, if I had six children I couldn't do all this for you". She believed in standing her children up in this world. One day I came home from school feeling very hypo, she simply lifted her newspaper and said, "test your urine and if it turns blue go to the pantry and help yourself". "It is really bad" I replied. "Then go to the pantry!" For years I thought that was mean of her to not get up and help me. Many years later, I realised or believed she was terrified and fixed to her seat. Hindsight is a great thing! I am now very grateful and thank her for her tough love as it made me independent and able to face life.

Aunty Jean was a Brown Owl and she took me away on a Brownie Pack Holiday to give my family a little respite. It was agreed as she was a nurse. For every step of my diabetes management she asked, "what did they teach you in hospital?" I knew what to do and I had a great time with the other brownies. Many years later Aunty Jean told us she worked on 'Men's Surgical Ward' and didn't really know a lot about managing a child with diabetes! It was great for me to go on the camp and mix with other children outside of those in my family, I didn't get a lot of invites to play at other children's houses. I suppose people were worried about me falling into a coma or collapsing during a hypo. I had just one good friend whose parents would take me caravanning and through her I met my husband. It just goes to show you don't need lots of friends in this life.

I went back to school after a month away. There were no allowances back then for disability and certainly no equality legislation or "reasonable adjustments". Mum was worried about carbohydrate counting at school and asked them if I may take sandwiches, but that was not allowed. I ended up having to cycle home for my lunch, often feeling a bit shaky as my bloods were low. I took the 11 plus but the first choice was for me to go to secondary modern. Mum explained to me that the doctor had told her stress would not be good for me. I was given a wicker basket and told I would be joining some lovely Methodist chapel girls. I recently found the basket in mum's barn and have kept it for old times' sake. It never stopped me and indeed spurred me on in later life to get a degree and master's degree with a distinction.

As a child I prayed for a cure until I read an article in the local paper describing a lady who had been cured. She had undergone a kidney and pancreas transplant and I immediately stopped praying! I didn't want to go through all of that in order to be cured. Maybe God had another plan.

My aunty Jean had delivered me into this world, when I arrived she said, "it's another nurse for the family". Well, it was the 1960's so everyone knew I was a girl! Gender roles were only just starting to be challenged. My mother, a teacher, said "No, she will be whatever she wants".

I never desired to be a nurse, I could see that my cousins were having a great time as student nurses. I hadn't learnt to drive and thought I fancied a flat of my own. I then thought I could be a nurse as I could at least give injections. Hospitals were a familiar place to me, so I applied for nurse training, much to my aunties and diabetes consultants delight. The consultant gave me an article that stated that diabetes girls make good nurses. I wish I still had it but I think I passed it on. Today, I am supporting a young woman with Type 1 who initially worked for me in an admin role but said she thought she could do my job. I thought she could do my job too, but I explained that she needed to be a registered nurse. She has achieved that now and is well on her way to becoming and diabetes specialist nurse (DSN).

When I started training I didn't want a fuss being made, so I always worked on a ward for a week or two then would ask the ward sister "Oh Sister, by the way, did the school of nursing let you know that I am type 1?" Panic would set in and I would then say
"no need to worry, I have been fine so far."
It was the routine that I used and it also worked well when I met my boyfriend, now husband. Still, I would then be sent to first breaks (which no one liked) and work 8 nights on duty in a stretch as 'they' felt it better. No evidence, but sister apparently knew best.
As a nurse I was working physically hard and I struggled on the ward to prevent hypos (not that people knew as I never said anything and I had found ways to eat and drink without people noticing).
I told my consultant I was leaving, she cancelled my notice and wrote away to buy a blood glucose meter for me. It was seventy pounds and dad paid her back. I wrote two cheques for £35 to my

dad on each pay day, but I later realized that they were never cashed.

There have been many changes to diabetes management over 50 years. Equipment has particularly changed. I started with the glass syringes but disposable needles given personally by my GP who had diagnosed me. My mother had asked how she would know when to change the needle, the reply was when it was blunt! Mother was very clear this would not be good enough for her Mary. Summer or winter, she always had a coat over her arm at GP appointments and was given a box of needles to smuggle out. In 1985 I went on a clinical trial to trial what is now a basal bolus regimen using an insulin pen. Clinical trials helped me engage with my condition and probably even saved me. I am very fortunate to have an insulin pump and sensor which is known as a closed loop. It is needed as night time hypos have been a real challenge for me for a number of years now. I always relied upon my husband to wake me until now as I never hear the alarms. My husband is pleased he can now get some sleep and not worry about me.

After qualifying as a nurse, I had my two children, first a son followed by a daughter. Pregnancy was one long concern ending with pre-eclampsia, hospital admissions, caesarean sections but two live special care babies. However, for the 1980s this wasn't bad. It was an emotional roller coaster throughout and I was sterilised with my second child aged 25 years old. I could not go through it again. After each child I chose to go back to nursing but on night duty. One night my friend and I during a quiet moment discussed what we would like to specialise in or what we might be when we grew up! She suggested I would make a great DSN and eventually that happened. I dreaded the interview as my own consultant was on the panel and I thought he would know I was far from a 'perfect' diabetic (I thought such people existed). Apparently, I was hilarious as I was the only candidate who listed all the different insulins, I was confident with this as I named all the ones I had taken. I was however worried about oral medications. I was also so flexible on the dietary question that they reminded me after the interview that a special occasion was not every day! I learnt so much from that consultant. At my appointments he used to go through my notes and say we have to keep you going forever Mary because you make a great DSN.

Being a DSN has been my life, setting up and improving services has been my passion. My happiest days were spent in Tower Hamlets, London, even though it took over two hours to commute to and from work. The service went from the worst to the best borough for diabetes outcome. The diabetes centre was named a beacon in the East End of London by a nursing journal.

Dream Trust

I first heard of the charity The DREAM Trust in 1998 when Diabetes UK published an article by Dr Sharad Pendsey called 'Where have all the girls gone?'
It told the story of how two girls died because their parents did not have enough money to pay for insulin. He, his wife and well-wishers set up the charity to provide free insulin for children.
 The words spoke directly me and I felt so thankful that I was born in England and was lucky enough to have free prescriptions.
I wondered how living and nursing in the UK, I might be able to help Dr Pendsey. Working as a DSN, I was used to representatives bringing samples into the office, often they went unused.
 I asked if I could send these unwanted gifts to India and Dr Pendsey wrote to thank me. Then one day he e-mailed to ask that I might go and give a talk to a girls' school in Ashford, Kent.

A pupil whose sister lived with type 1 Diabetes had read the same article and put forward The DREAM Trust to become their school charity of the year. I went to the school assembly to give a talk about Dr Pendsey's work and I found myself saying how I would love to go there, meet the children and see the charity in action for myself.

We arranged to go at the end of 1999. The staff met my husband and I as we came off the flight and they put garlands around my head. It was a very warm welcome and we were the first visitors from overseas to visit the Trust. We visited patients on the hospital ward, in diabetes clinic and went out on home visits. I gave a talk to the children and health care professionals. The talk to the health care professionals was important as many were puzzled as to why Dr Pendsey should have saved the girls as they feared for their future. I gave a talk about how I got diabetes aged 10 years, how I studied at school and became a diabetes educator, married had two children of my own and then continued to work. The story inspired them that their own children could live a life worth living, despite diabetes. The women in the audience though thought my husband was the most amazing for allowing me to go to work!

I have remained a supporter ever since. Dr & Mrs Pendsey have stayed with us in the UK when he had a lecture to give and he met up with Jenny Hirst, the founder of Insulin Dependent Diabetes Trust (IDDT) who's member's sponsor the children. We met up in Dubai at an International Diabetes Conference where we supported him giving a DREAM Trust lecture. We have since returned to Nagpur to visit the clinic and meet the children we sponsor. It is a privilege to be a part of this charity and see the support grow. We encouraged others to go and visit the clinic from this Lucy Todd founded The Pendsey Trust, a UK support for the DREAM Trust.
We returned to India in 2012 and the Trust had grown and here was our report.

Thursdays are Dream Trust clinic days. The children arrive (some having. travelled for 3-4 hours) and are met by the Nursing Sister who collects their empty insulin bottles and she takes a blood test for HbA1c. Next the Diabetes Specialist Educator, Seema, a dietitian, makes a note of the child's weight after they have happily hopped on the scales. They know the routine well and are clearly happy in the diabetes clinic. Seema talks to the children about how they are coping with their diabetes and school or college. She listens to their mothers or fathers concerns or sisters, who come to support the older children. One young type 1 mother came proudly with her baby daughter.

Seema makes a note of what insulin they take. It is unit 40 strength and tends to be soluble (quick acting) and Isophane (intermediate). They mix the insulin in the syringe night and morning but tend to need some soluble insulin middle of the day because their diet is mainly carbohydrate based and lacking in protein. One young teenage man wanted to gain muscles, but exercise alone was not helping, Seema recommended he buy some nuts from the stalls on the street as milk was far too expensive for his family. One mother cried as she said her neighbours wanted her to stop the insulin in favour of herbal remedies as her child cried at injection times. She was encouraged to be strong and do the right thing. The little girl concerned saw her mum was upset and made a promise to have her insulin without too much of a fuss, she then shook hands with Seema to keep her promise.

Once the HbA1c result was available Dr Pendsey decided if the insulin needed adjusting. The results for the children in the clinic that day were between 7 - 8%, which was impressive given the

children did not usually blood glucose test at this time. HbA1c, a history of the child's food/exercise, clinical experience and the child's weight helped with dose adjustment recommendations. Hypos have to be kept to a minimum as an ambulance and hospitalisation remains too expensive for many families. Five of the children joined
a research programme which gave them a free blood glucose meter and enough strips to test twice a day. The research continued for 18 months and evaluated a number of questions: if HbA1c improved and if this is maintained, who tests and who declines to test regularly. 250 children were recruited to the research project.

While we were there my husband presented the 50th bicycle the Dream Trust had provided and I gave the educational sponsorship for school uniform and books to another child. This helps the children to do well at school as when they are older it is hoped they will be able to start paying for some and then all of their insulin. One young man has done so well he now buys his own insulin and sponsors a child. Thanks and gratitude indeed!

We visited three families on our home visits. The families met us at landmarks near to their homes and guided us to their home. The first child had type 1 diabetes and Downs Syndrome. She went to the local school but could not read or write. She had a sister and was very friendly, once she got over her initial
shyness of strangers coming to her three roomed home.
Her father had recently found work for the government. They had paid for a fridge to keep the insulin in as a previous doctor had not been happy to prescribe insulin without a fridge.

The next child was an only child. Both the mother and father worked. The father was a night watchman but earned only enough money for the rental of one room. Mother had two jobs cooking which meant she paid for some electricity and food. They kept the child's insulin next to the Hindu worship area. They had no fridge.

The final visit was to a five-year-old boy who lived with his parents, grandparents and two sisters in two rooms. Water for all the families was a tap outside and they had to store water, as it is only available for an hour each day. The little boy had just joined the Dream Trust and his HbA1c was 15%. The family had only just heard about Dr Pendsey and were struggling to buy insulin. He was their only son and clearly mothered by everyone but even for him the money for sufficient insulin was too much. He became our sponsored child.

Before we left we celebrated World Diabetes Day with at least 150 in the audience. Never in my career have I seen so many children with type 1 diabetes in one room before. We in the UK could learn so much about diabetes care and support. I gave a motivational speech about living with type 1 diabetes and how diabetes care has improved since the discovery of insulin. Others including three of the children gave speeches telling how they had overcome living with the challenges of diabetes. The afternoon concluded with a buffet curry.

Our memories of the amazing work of the staff and trustees of the Dream Trust and the testimony of the children have served to motivate us to continue to support the charity by highlighting its essential work. We fundraise to make sure even more children with type 1 diabetes can be saved. I have remained in touch with the staff, children and joined the Pendsey Trust to support the children's insulin education. It is easier nowadays with e-mails and social media to keep in touch.

I am a lady of a certain age and have retired but returned to nursing. Having been a DSN and nursed in city, town and village, I feel I have so much experience and the passion to help people with

diabetes. I enjoy educating the health care professionals that I now work with in the largest and smallest surgeries in Stevenage. It is now, rightly, fashionable not to judge or tell patients off in clinics. For me I never could be like that as I have had my own struggles. I have always asked people how they are, used this approach and
found it leads to great success for patients and it gives me such satisfaction.

I look forward, God willing, to receiving my Diabetes UK medal, which is awarded to people who have lived with diabetes for 50 years. I have had my eyes on this for many, many years. I never anticipated COVID-19 and so pray I will still get this. I want it for my doctors and nurses, for me and my family, especially mum and my late dad, but most of all, to show the children in India and everyone I meet that you can have a life worth living with type 1 diabetes.

Top tip for parents: it is not your fault that your child has diabetes, encourage and support them to be independent. Your child does not want you to be sad.

Tip for a person with diabetes: Just do your best, work with your team and find the best diabetes team for you.

You can learn about the 50 year medal Diabetes UK award at the link below, medals are also awarded after 60, 70 and 80 years.
https://www.diabetes.org.uk/about_us/medals

To find out more about Mary and to see her photo's, check out our website at www.typeawesome.co.uk

Chapter 9

"I can actually play a full 90-minute game now without having to do anything with my diabetes."

Tilly-Rose Dade

Tilly-Rose is only 13 years old but has lived with Type 1 most of her life. Tilly has a promising career as a footballer ahead of her. She is a very active young lady and works tirelessly everyday towards her dream of being a professional female footballer. Tilly plays for Norwich City Elite team and tells us about her new pump and how it has changed her life, as well as how she manages diabetes around her football schedule.

My diagnosis was June, 2011, I was four years old. I had a few problems when I was really young but at age 4 I started losing a lot of weight. My Mum had to put me back in nappies after I had previously been dry. I would also get very tired. One day, we went on a family trip to the strawberry "pick your own" farm, I ate the whole of my punnet but then said that the strawberries made me feel really good. My Mum wondered why I would say that, most 4-year olds would just say that the strawberries were yummy.

My Mum had been taking me back and forth to the Doctors for a while as I had been unwell for some time, but the Doctor just kept saying I had a virus. A few days after the strawberry farm trip and I fell unconscious during a car journey, I had been drinking a lot of juice that morning. I was rushed into hospital and it was discovered that my blood sugars were extremely high, this is where my story with diabetes starts.

I was too young to understand what was happening or what was wrong with me but I do remember all the injections I had to have back then. My Mum tells me that she gave me my insulin injection for the first time 3 hours after I was diagnosed with Type One Diabetes. I didn't like the injections and I would cry.

My parents were devastated, I think my diagnosis turned their world upside down because suddenly they had to learn so much about how to keep me not just alive but also keep me well.

I was eventually well enough to come home and we learnt how to fit diabetes into our lives. Mum had to test me in the night and I remember I used to suffer really stubborn low hypo's, I was force fed whilst half asleep quite a few times. I must have been very worrying for her. I know one time my blood sugar was 0.9, apparently, I was non-responsive. I think that is the lowest I have ever been.

As I got older I began to learn more about diabetes and about my care. A whole new set of words came into my vocabulary, words like hypo, hyper, ketones, ratios, insulin, bolus, basal and diabetes. I learnt what these words were and what I had to do to keep well. I had between 8 and 10 injections and blood tests a day for the first three years following my diagnosis. I just got used to them and eventually I stopped crying because there wasn't really anything else I could do. I had accepted that I needed them. I have always shown a keen interest in sport, especially football. I knew that if I did not do my injections then I could not play football because I wouldn't be well enough. Not playing football makes me sad. I must admit though, back in those days my blood sugars were like a rollercoaster, I used to have very low hypo's and very high hypers. It was very hard to keep me in the target range.

My family and I came to accept my diagnosis, it wasn't going to go away and living in denial is not possible. We respect my diabetes now and know I must monitor myself regularly and give myself insulin but life doesn't stop. As a family we continued to do everything we would normally do, including going on holiday, going on days out, going to parties, eating everything at the buffet, going on school trips (including the residential ones) and as I am very sporty, I joined in a wide range of sporting activities. Football is my favourite sport though and nothing is going to stop me from playing football. Diabetes does not control my life, I work hard to control my diabetes.

My family are amazing and very supportive, they keep me upbeat and don't let me stay down for long. My hospital team are brilliant and are always there for me when and if I need them, always professional and full of supportive advice. I don't think there is a situation they haven't come across before and they are always giving me tips. My school is fantastic, they never leave me out and they always make sure I can take part in all the activities they offer, including the school trips.

Dreamflight

I was nine when I was offered an amazing opportunity. Dreamflight are a UK based registered charity who take young children with serious illnesses or disabilities on a holiday of a lifetime to Florida, without their families. My Consultant at Norwich and Norfolk University Hospital nominated me for this once in a lifetime trip to Orlando. I boarded a 747 with the other children who had chronic illnesses or disabilities, and all the people looking after us were Doctors, Nurses and other medical professionals. I knew that I had support with my diabetes care if I needed it both on the plane and throughout the trip. Even the flight out there was so much fun because they made it like a big party. Also, when we got to Orlando, we got on a convoy of coaches to go to the hotel and the Police close off the streets and give us a VIP escort to our hotel.

The week I spent in Florida was fantastic. We went to all the attractions, including Walt Disney's Magic Kingdom, Universal

Studios, Islands of Adventure, Sea World but the highlight was going to Discovery Cove where we got to swim with dolphins. Dolphins are wonderful creatures and I will always treasure the memory of swimming with them.

I had an amazing time and made new friends. I think going on a trip like this at a young age made me more independent and increased my confidence. I was also with other children who live with serious health conditions, so I didn't feel alone or different. I could talk to others about things like managing my healthcare at school, the effects of my condition on my family, how I feel about repeat hospital visits and how I manage my condition around my life. I didn't feel like the odd one out, in fact, on that trip it was quite the norm to have a chronic and serious health condition, that alone feels less isolating even though there were people there with a wide range of conditions and disabilities, not just Type One Diabetes.

Pump and freedom

I was about 7 when we looked into getting me an insulin pump. I wasn't too keen on a tubed pump, I didn't want a reminder I have diabetes or to get the tubing tangled or the cannula to pull off when I was playing sports. So, I chose the Omnipod, we decided it was the best pump for me out of the ones that were available at the time. I didn't have to worry about the tubing getting tangled in my football kit. The Omnipod gave me freedom from so many injections as it was just one needle with a cannula in that needed changing every 3 days. I also gained funding at the same time for a Dexcom, which continually read my glucose levels and alerts me or Mum if I go low. It worked quite well for me and Mum was less anxious because
she could see what my levels were on her phone, even when I was at school or at my friends' houses. Mum could check my levels whilst she was watching me play football without having to pull me

out of the game. Omnipod and Dexcom's aren't a cure though of course, and unfortunately, I was still having really bad hypo's, some of them resulting in a hospital admission. I hated how the hypo's were affecting me at school and at football and just couldn't get them under control.

In 2019, my diabetes team told me about a new pump called Medtronic 670g and a CGM called Guardian 3, they offered me funding for both and suggested to me that it was a better way to manage my diabetes as it can slow down or stop insulin if the Guardian 3 sensed I was dropping too low. It did appear to have the ability to help me, but at the same time it seemed a bit daunting to think about a whole new way of managing diabetes. I remember when I started on Omnipod there was a lot to learn, a lot of adjustments to make, ratio's to change and different basal time blocks . I was also concerned that the 670g has tubing and that might take some getting used to, especially with all the sport I do. With the support of my family and my medical team, I went away and looked into the 670g a bit more and learnt that it is semi-automatic, the pump can communicate with the CGM and make automatic adjustments. I decided to give it all try, after all, it was just an initial trial at first to see how I liked it and no commitment was needed to do the trial. I loved it and I can honestly say it changed my life for the better. If my bloods start to rise, the pump gives me more insulin until they are within target levels. If the pump detects I am going low it can reduce or suspend insulin which prevents hypo's. This would be a game changer for my football and this set up made a massive change to my life. I spent so much more time in range, I improved my HbA1c and I was even sleeping better because of the pump. My teachers even noticed that my attendance was better because I am having less time off school, less time at hospital and I am even concentrating better and this will only reflect in my results.

My football has improved as I no longer have to worry about hypo's or have to stop playing every 10-15 minutes to test my blood. I can simply get on with the game or my training, knowing that if I go low my pump will deal with it and also warn me. In the past when I was at football, if my blood sugar was too high or too low it would really affect me on the pitch. I would get so frustrated when I needed to come off to test or have sugary drinks and snacks. Now, I can just play the whole game and it is brilliant. I can actually play a full 90-minute game now without having to do anything with my diabetes. It is amazing. I do however still take a lot of glucotabs to football, just in case. A lot of good diabetes management is down to thinking about what you might need and making sure you have everything.

Another little thing I have to keep myself safe is a medic alert bracelet. Although I now have the pump and CGM attached to me, the medic alert is an extra re-assurance if an emergency was to occur. My own club, Norwich City, are aware of my diabetes but there could be times when people are standing in or we are playing away and the medic might not know I have diabetes. Not only that, but the medic alert links to my medical files so my family can be confident and reassured that any information the medical team need is just a quick phone call away. My Mum has said that me having my medic alert bracelet has made it easier for her to start letting go and letting me walk home from school with my friends, get the bus into town, have sleepovers and just generally be a teenager. Medic alert offer a wide range of bracelets and jewellery now, so there is sure to be one that you like. I have a sports band one, it is perfect for sports and looks good too. It is just an extra way to keep myself safe now I am at an age where I want more independence.

I currently play football with Norwich City Girls Football Academy, I am also an England Centre for Excellence player. I played in the nationals last year and my dream is to one day represent England in the women's football world cup. I hope that one day I can be a professional female footballer, it is all I want to do when I leave school. I know for sure that diabetes is not going to stop me from achieving my dream.

Tilly's top tip "Control your diabetes, don't let it control you"
Tilly's top tip to parents "Get a medic alert for your child"

We have since learnt that Tilly had some issues over lockdown and was quite ill, as a result, she is not currently using the 670G but we are pleased to hear she is doing much better and has returned to football. We wish Tilly-Rose all the best for the future and look forward to cheering her on when she plays in the world cup final!

Get a medic-alert at:
https://www.medicalert.org.uk/

To keep up to date with Tilly-Rose and see some photos, check out
www.typeawesome.co.uk

Chapter 10

"My cousin saved my life, even though he had died 58 years earlier!"

Rebecca Redmond

Rebecca is Canadian, she was diagnosed with Type 1 Diabetes when she was 17. She also suffers from Mental Health issues, but she does not let anything get in her way despite these challenges. Rebecca home-schools her son, runs a blog to support others with Type 1 and Mental Health problems, and volunteers for organisations that support people with diabetes. She is also an ambassador for Insulet, which involves sitting on panels and other media posts; she even travelled to Barcelona to sit on a panel earlier this year. Rebecca has a famous ancestral cousin who saved her life and those of many millions or even billions of diabetics around the world. Rebecca is a relative of the legend Sir Frederick Grant Banting.

Please note that Canada does not have an NHS like the UK, unfortunately, even Fred Banting's cousin does not have access to free insulin. Diabetes supplies in Canada can be very expensive, as is insurance which does not always cover the costs. Also, some products mentioned in this chapter may not be available in the UK. It is worth bearing this in mind when reading Rebecca's story.

I grew up knowing about a very famous person in my ancestry. I have fond memories of my Grandmother talking about this incredible man and of how proud she was of everything he had achieved. This man (a distant cousin to me) had made remarkable achievements in many areas of his life, but one discovery that would go on to save lives of millions of people around the world. My distant cousin is Sir Frederick Grant Banting, the man who discovered a way to isolate insulin and use it to treat diabetic patients. My cousin is the man who made it possible for us to say "I live with diabetes."

I too am incredibly proud to be related to such a generous and amazing man, I obviously grew up knowing Banting's story and I knew a bit about diabetes and insulin. I was aware that prior to my cousin's discovery, diabetes was always fatal. At best people lived a couple of years, but had blindness, amputations, organ failure and no quality of life. Death was the only escape and the only certainty.
My cousin was a doctor and scientific researcher, he realized that if he could isolate animal insulin and inject it into humans, their blood sugars might lower. Just 15 months after this idea, he had injected his first patients successfully and they went on to live largely normal lives.

My cousin's discovery became even more relevant to me when just before my 18th birthday, I was diagnosed with Type 1 Diabetes myself. It came as a bit of a shock, despite our family often talking about Banting's work in diabetes no one had experienced type 1 diabetes themselves in our family. Diagnosis was a real surprise, I had no genetic markers or other illnesses to note. My cousin saved my life, even though he had died 58 years earlier!

All of a sudden, I could understand the importance of his discovery on a totally different level. I was all too aware of just how remarkable his achievement was, without him I might not have seen my 18th birthday and certainly wouldn't have made my 19th. Just what this man had done was now much more personal, he had not only saved millions of lives around the world, but he had saved my life. I am sure my family were even more grateful for Fred Banting than they had ever been!

Prior to my cousin's discovery, people diagnosed with Type 1 were effectively given a painful death sentence. The human body cannot survive long without insulin, within hours of having no insulin in the body dramatic events take place that put life at risk. Any efforts to treat diabetes prior to 1921 just prolonged life for a short length of time in which the person had no quality of life. Eventually, the patient would die from starvation, severe malnutrition and multiple organ failure, often within months. Anyone who managed to survive longer would have multiple organ failure, amputations, blindness and generally feel so weak they wouldn't be able to get out of bed. So, after my own diagnosis, I became even more aware of the extent of the importance of my cousin's discovery. My cousin not only saved the lives of so many people worldwide who live with Type 1 diabetes, but he also gave them their life back and made it possible that they could achieve whatever they wanted and follow their dreams, just as long as they have the insulin.

Today, life expectancy for people living with Type 1 Diabetes in the western world is almost the same as everyone else. Type 1 is no reason why a child, teenager or young person should not be playing sport, joining a school production, taking part in extreme sports, going to parties, having sleepovers, going on a date, go to school, college or university, going backpacking or travelling around the world or even eating chocolate cake! We just have to make more plans and prepare more than someone without diabetes, but as long as we keep using the insulin my cousin developed properly, we can lead full and happy lives. Thank you, Cousin Frederick!

As I was almost 18 at diagnosis, it was a bit complicated for me to learn all about my condition and how to best manage it. I think 17 is a difficult age to be diagnosed, as I was older I already had a lot of freedom and my parents (although they are wonderfully supportive) were not involved with the day to day care because I was already spending a lot of time away from them preparing to go to university, socializing with friends, and so on. Even now, when I visit Mom, she sometimes forgets to remind me 20 minutes before dinner is ready, so I end up doing my insulin late! At almost 18, I was too old for the juvenile team, I missed out on the meet ups with peers, and going away on diabetes camp. I was placed in an adult's diabetes clinic and had to go on learning sessions with people who had Type 2 Diabetes, which I am sure you all know is quite different! I did not get the opportunity to meet other people who had Type 1 for many, many years. In fact, it was nearly two decades before I met another Type 1 in the flesh. It was quite an isolating time for me, but I just had to get on with it and do my best.

Over the 20 years following my diagnosis, I lived with the highs and lows, the frustration, and the pain. I had no one else to share these with, although my husband and my family were incredibly supportive. I had no one else to talk to who was going through the same as me, no one who just got it and totally knew how it feels. I participated in a JDRF event, the year of my 20th diaversary, spending the entire day with people who also have Type 1. I felt so much love and support, much less alone and a lot more understood. I could not believe the depths of community out there; I also could not believe I had not tapped into it before that day. I highly recommend anyone dealing with Type 1 get involved in their local Type 1 community for support, it is so important to meet other people who understand exactly what you are going through. This advice extends to parents too, parents need support and need to know other parents of children with Type 1. Do not let it take you or
your child 20 years to get involved!

In June 2009, my life changed again. I had received another diagnosis. I was pregnant! How was I going to manage my diabetes, pregnancy and a child? I had an awful lot of concerns. I was classed as a high-risk pregnancy and my general practitioner referred me to a specialist. My husband was over the moon, he had always wanted to be a father. I however was very scared. I imagined that scene from Steel Magnolias, in which Julia Roberts portrays a character with Type 1 and is found unconscious in the kitchen, with pots boiling over and the baby crying on the floor. I was worried about burdening a child with my chronic illnesses and I had doubts I would be a good mother.

My doctors kept emphasizing the importance of tight control throughout the pregnancy. I had weekly appointments, lots of extra tests, procedures and trips to specialists. I had to test my blood every 2 hours, even in the night. I had to record everything on a chart for my endocrinologist, that included all the test results, injections, carbs, hypos, hypers, ketones. Everything! I also suffer with body dysmorphia, and I struggled with my mental health. I gained nearly 100 pounds, even though I was pregnant this did not seem good to me and negatively impacted my mental health.

I did find a lot of positives too. I had lived with diabetes for 10 years at this stage and I had always feared needles (even before I was diagnosed). I had never properly learned to inject myself, but when I was pregnant, I had no option but to learn; it wasn't just about me anymore but about the life that was growing inside of me. A rite of passage for diabetics is injecting an orange for practice, one I was denied at diagnosis due to been sent to learn with the Type 2 patients. My new diabetes team took me right back to the basics and I started by finally injecting an orange. This was not just a physical thing I had to overcome, but a mental one too. I got used to
seeing needles and the process of injecting. After the orange, it

was time to start properly injecting myself. I injected my pregnant belly and used the correct injecting technique, this was a huge moment for me. As I was now injecting properly, and regularly, my HbA1c improved and was the best it has ever been. It remained at or around 6% (42) the whole way through my pregnancy! Another plus was the fact I learned about correction doses, what they are and how to calculate and do them. I had not learned this when I was first diagnosed. Because I had been lumped with T2 patients I obtained little information about insulin and how to administer it. Of course, correction doses also helped me to get better control. Overall, my pregnancy was problem free even though my baby was born 4 weeks prematurely. I did displace a hip during childbirth, which was painful and made it difficult for the first few weeks at home with a new-born. Overall, I was pleased to have given birth to a healthy baby boy. All this despite the Doctors initially telling me that I would have problems in pregnancy due to diabetes and it might even be impossible for me to carry a healthy baby to term. Today, that baby is a healthy and happy 10-year-old.

I struggled to breastfeed, something I was unaware was typical of T1D mothers. At the hospital, I had to supplement his feeds with formula milk because his blood sugar needed to be stabilized. I felt guilty, ill equipped and like I had failed him. At 5 months old, my son was diagnosed with a milk allergy so had to switch to soy formula. I also learned more about T1D mothers having problems lactating and increased hypoglycaemia. It was not my fault! I was incredibly relieved. Do not let Type 1 ruin your baby's first months, babies can still thrive on formula options.

When my son was young, I was his primary care giver. I feared my blood sugars going low whilst home alone with him, so I admit I used to purposefully let my sugars run a bit high, or coast along to avoid this.

By the time, my son was 18 months old, we had explained to him about Type 1 and showed him how he could help Mommy. He was able to help me test and knew where my treatments were kept so he could always grab me some fast-acting sugary snacks if I was low. I was however still very scared of going too low while I was on my own with him, so preferred to run a bit high in order to avoid lows. It was a difficult time but extremely rewarding to see this young life I had created develop into a loving young boy.

I find it interesting that pregnancy motivated me to care for myself. My baby depended on me, but I still struggled with managing diabetes. I always put him and his health first. The saying "fasten your seatbelt before helping others" comes to mind here, though it was not what I practiced. As my son grew older, he showed an interest in my diabetes and would hug me when he saw me struggling to inject. We also trained him about what to do if ever he ever found me unconscious. He knew how to call 911, what to say and even knew how to administer glucagon, should it ever be needed.

My son was taught all about our famous cousin Banting, he knew that one of his ancestors had made the discovery and that discovery was keeping Mommy alive. I once wore a CGM for a week, a trial offered by my then diabetes clinic. My son was fascinated that he could see my blood sugars and that I didn't need to finger prick to check my numbers. I didn't keep the CGM as unfortunately, without free healthcare in Canada, it was out of our financial reach at that time.

We learned about insulin pumps together. I had not been interested in having one because I did not want to make my invisible illness visible at that time. I was worried about having something attached to me 24/7. My then 5-year-old said, "if it could help you Mommy, you should have it." I could not really argue with that, so I enrolled in the pump classes my province's government required to get funding for a pump, in Ontario. I had to decide which pump I wanted and provide three consecutive Hba1c tests to get the pump. However, I missed a test due to a cancer diagnosis and treatment. Receiving the pump was delayed. Thankfully, I had two surgeries for that, but the pump had been put to the back of my mind and I did not pursue it.

Before my pregnancy, we never had glucagon in the house. We simply could not justify the cost. It is expensive and usually sits in the fridge until it expires. Even after a seriously bad hypo prior to my pregnancy, we struggled to navigate appropriating the funds for additional (and seemingly non-essential) diabetes equipment. Pregnancy changed my attitude on this, now I was responsible for another life and I needed to be more responsible about my health. We decided glucagon was important and hoped we would not ever need it. Fingers crossed, it would just expire in the fridge, but at least we would have it if the worst were to happen. We always made sure we had enough money for glucagon, keeping one in my bag and an expired one in the fridge "just in case." Thankfully, we now have insurance coverage for it, which helps!

It is hard for loved ones to administer glucagon as it is a different procedure than the one we are used to, not only that, but if it ever needs to be used loved ones will be panicking. My family expressed their concerns about not having the confidence to administer glucagon if it was ever needed, so we started looking into alternatives. It is amazing the speed that diabetes technology is making, we learnt that a new type of glucagon is available called Baqsimi. Baqsimi is basically glucagon that does not require preparing and injecting, instead, it is a nasal powder and does not even have to be inhaled because obviously the person would be unconscious if it were needed. I discussed the possibility of using
Baqsimi instead of glucagon with my family, thankfully they agreed it was a great invention and we were all pleased when it became

available in Canada in December 2019. Thankfully, my insurance covered the cost and we sat down and learned how to administer it properly. My husband and son were so relieved, it was so much easier than injecting glucagon. They are now confident they can use it if it is needed. My son said, "it is easier to help Mommy and not be afraid." Thankfully, most of the cost of Baqsimi is covered by our insurance but the re-assurance it gives my family is priceless.

When new Flash Glucose Monitoring (FGM) technology became available in Canada, I leapt at the opportunity to use it. This was fantastic for me because I did not have to finger prick to get blood, which meant I would test more. My son loved it because he could scan me to see what my blood sugars were and then he liked to dictate to me what he thought the next step was. We then moved to a new house in a new city, it meant a new diabetes team for me. This seemed like the perfect opportunity for a new start with an insulin pump. I must say that my motivation behind getting a pump was like my motivation was in pregnancy, I did it for my son. I did it because my son deserves his mother to be as healthy as she can be. I did it because I had to learn to fasten my own seatbelt before I could help others. I now use an Omnipod, a tubeless pump with no wires, and can easily hide the pod behind clothing, if I do not want my invisible illness visible. With my (now) Dexcom CGM and my Omnipod, I am cyborg Mom! We regularly joke about my robot body parts. My son has learned to use the pump PDM, and if I am driving for example and need an adjustment, he knows how to do it for me via the Personal Diabetes Manager (PDM - the handset that controls the pump).

Pregnancy and parenting are not easy but throwing Type 1 into the mix brings a lot more considerations. It is a road I am incredibly pleased I travelled down and overcame the challenges of, because bringing up a child is so rewarding! Pregnancy changed my life for the better, not only that, but it allowed me to finally take better care of my diabetes.

These days I can be found at home with my son, who is home-schooled. I always have a pen or paintbrush in my hand. I wanted to raise awareness and offer support to others living with both Type 1 Diabetes and mental illness, so I set up a blog called Dead Pancreas Anxiety. I blog there with an unapologetic truthfulness and a dose of humour. I hope I am giving those in that group a voice within the diabetes community. I want to change perceptions of what is considered "normal" and now advocate on a global scale, hopefully erasing stigma whilst doing so. My connection to Sir Frederick Banting and my own experiences with Type One Diabetes are the drive behind my diabetes advocacy. I am now an ambassador for Insulet, which gave me the opportunity to travel to Barcelona and speak about my experiences with diabetes. I have since enjoyed many other opportunities to share my experiences. I met some amazing people in Barcelona who live with Type 1, this was a fantastic way for me to get support and hopefully help others too.

I am passionately creative and have always enjoyed art. Maybe I inherited this from my famous cousin because he too was an artist. I recently re-created one of his pieces to raise awareness for JDRF Canada. I am so grateful I can use my talents to help raise vital funds that help to improve life for people with type one. Now, I am working on an art piece that will be created using my Omnipod pods from my first year of pumping. I hope it will raise awareness of diabetes, but it also provided me a creative outlet. Look out for that one!

I am tremendously grateful for the Type One community, for my famous cousin, and for the new people I continue to meet because diabetes every one of them inspires me. I am grateful for my wonderful husband and son, for that pregnancy, which helped me turn my life and diabetes management around. I would like to continue my cousin's work by advocating for people living with diabetes, to raise awareness about the need to make insulin more affordable and accessible, helping everyone who needs insulin achieve sustainable access to it.

Rebecca's top tip: Get involved in your T1 community, you need support from others going through it.

Rebecca's blog is:

http://www.deadpancreasanxiety.com/

To find out more about Rebecca and to see her photos, including the one where her cousin Banting grew up, go to **www.typeawesome.co.uk**

Chapter 11

"We are JDRF. We won't stop until we create a world without Type 1 Diabetes."

JDRF

Juvenile Diabetes Research Foundation (JDRF) are a global charity striving to eradicate Type 1 Diabetes, by funding research into a cure and then identifying those at risk of developing it and preventing the onset of diabetes.

JDRF are aiming to do this by:

- Funding world class research, which is approved and administered by international research programme to cure, treat and prevent type 1 diabetes

- Ensure research continues to move forward and treatments are delivered to patients in a timely manner

- Give support and advocacy to people with Type 1 and their loved ones

Here are some interesting facts about JDRF:

- JDRF are currently funding over 500 research projects globally and is supporting more than 70 clinical trials. Internationally, over £1.5 billion in research funding has been awarded by JDRF.

- Research is only funded if it could transform the lives of people with type 1, improving treatments until the day a cure is found and after that, can Type 1 be prevented?

- JDRF work with partner organisations as the collaborative value brings us closer to a cure much quicker

- JDRF do not fund projects aimed at treating or curing other types of diabetes, only research that improves life for people with t1.

JDRF fund research that aims to:

- Improve management of Type 1 Diabetes

- Cure Type 1 Diabetes biologically

- Prevent Type 1 Diabetes

Let's take a look at some of the current projects JDRF are funding.

Improving Management

Some scientists are looking into ways to improve management of Type 1, if treatment options can be improved this will make life easier for the person who lives with Type 1 until a cure can be found.

Drug Trials - Professor John Petrie, University of Glasgow

Professor Petrie is a global leader in diabetes research, his team at Glasgow are testing semaglutide and, dapagliflozin drugs that are thought to improve blood glucose levels in adults with Type 1 Diabetes. The drugs would both need to be taken as a combination therapy along with some insulin injections, the aim of the treatment is to reduce hba1c in adult patients to 7% or less, with some of the management involved in diabetes being eliminated.

It is thought that used together, dapagliflozin and semaglutide can reduce the fluctuations in blood glucose and in turn this will improve the quality of life for people living with type 1. As blood sugars will not fluctuate high, the potential for long term complications is also reduced.

Glucose Responsive Insulin (GRI) or Smart Insulin

Glucose Responsive Insulin, also known as Smart Insulin, is insulin which only activates when it is needed. GRI would allow a person to take insulin once a day and it will activate when required and any access insulin would dissolve or melt. Basically, the smart insulin would automatically respond to changing blood glucose levels and "switch on" when needed. Smrt insulin would work in the same way as pancreas works in a person without diabetes. Several companies and universities are working on developing smart insulin, including options of it being taken by once a day injection, tablet, capsule or even a patch.

GRI sounds like an absolute dream - blood sugars would always be in range, there would be no lows, no highs, no injection or cannulas, no blood testing or CGM's, no risk of DKA and no anxiety! Unfortunately though, research is still in the very early stages so it is likely to be many years yet until it becomes available. Many of the research projects are 5 - 10 years away from human trial. It does sound promising though, especially one of the smart insulin patches that also has beta cells!

Artificial Pancreas Research

An artificial pancreas is a piece of technology that would be worn externally on the body to deliver automatic basal insulin delivery (via a cannula), which reduces the time and effort that is currently dedicated to managing Type 1 diabetes. An insulin pump and a Continuous Glucose Monitor (CGM) are combined and communicate with each other, the pump will detect glucose levels and adjust insulin doses accordingly. The device uses a specialized computer programme called an algorithm to monitor and adjust insulin continuously, which helps keep the person within range.

The Medtronic 670G is the current device that does this, it takes away some of the work involved in managing diabetes and it is very good and preventing highs and hypo's. The algorithm behind the Medtronic 670g clinical trial was funded by JDRF. Many users of the 670G hail that it is like having a cure, although it is a giant leap forward in management, it is still lacking some functions that mean the user has no input at all. For example, the 670G algorithm cannot calculate and adjust insulin levels at mealtimes, so the user must manually carb count and enter the carb content into the pump manually, the pump will then deliver the insulin.

JDRF are funding research and clinical trials into artificial pancreas studies across the world as they believe better ways to manage Type 1 are a short-term aim, whilst the cure will come in the longer term. JDRF realise that patients need looking after now and until a cure is discovered.

One recipient of an artificial pancreas grant is University of Cambridge researcher, Professor Roman Hovorka, who is a specialist in creating computer programmes that mimic how the human body works. Professor Hovorka developed an artificial pancreas system called CamAPS FX that can be runs on an android app, it was launched in 2020. The launch of this app is a milestone towards using artificial pancreas technology for everyone with diabetes.

The app, CamAPS FX, communicates with an insulin pump and a CGM and has a very complicated algorithm which can automatically deliver insulin. Professor Hovorka hopes the app will become available on the NHS and it can take over management of the condition which people with Type 1 will find especially beneficial at night when blood sugars can go low in their sleep. The app can communicate with diabetes management software and other technologies, such as diasend, which in turn enables diabetes professionals to provide more personalized care to their patients.

The CamAPS FX app was 13 years in clinical research, it was funded by JDRF and several other organisations including Diabetes UK, National Institute for Health Research and the Leona M and Harry B Helmsley Charitable Trust. It is also the very first artificial pancreas system that is licenced for use in pregnancy and very young children, as infants as young as 12 months can use it.

Professor Hovorka himself has stated that he is aiming for his research to "alleviate the ever-present burden of type 1 and improve health outcomes" whilst JDRF state 'this app is a major innovation and a significant milestone on the road to a fully automated and interoperable artificial pancreas."

Potential Biological Cures

Type 1 diabetes happens when the immune system wrongly attacks the beta cells in the pancreas, which make insulin. The cells then become damaged and insulin can no longer be produced. Science is investigating different ways that the damaged beta cells can be either replaced or regenerated so that pancreas can produce insulin again.

Growing beta cells from stem cells - Dr Rocio Sancho, Kings College London

Dr Sancho and her team are hoping to develop a new way to make beta cells from stem cells whilst also gaining a better understanding of the conditions that make this process happen. Beta cells will be created from stem cells, then implanted into mice to see if they can produce insulin and if, if they can make enough insulin for their demands. It is hoped that this research can contribute towards developing a treatment where beta cells are transplanted into patients with Type 1, enabling them to make their own insulin again.

It is thought that Dr Sancho's research will provide a better understanding of type 1 and how it can be treated with stem cells. It could improve knowledge of how many stem cells are needed to grow the required amount of beta cells. This research could be combined with research on how to prevent the immune system attacking the transplanted stem cells, such as encapsulation or drug therapy. Dr Sancho's research could lead to a world where people with type 1 diabetes do not need to inject, or the number of injections needed is reduced. I'm sure you agree, this sounds very encouraging!

Encapsulation

Insulin producing cells can already be transplanted into someone with Type 1 Diabetes, but the problem is that the immune system kills them off again (just like what happened when the person first developed T1D). Anti-rejections drugs can be given to help overcome this, but these in themselves can cause serious problems and have nasty side effects. Even if cells are successfully transplanted and anti-rejection drugs are taken with no problems, research has formerly found that the insulin making cells will not make insulin forever, so the benefits are only seen as temporary. This then means the risks associated with transplantation and anti-rejection drugs far outweighs any benefits, and as the insulin cells don't last long it places a higher demand on organ donors and there are currently not enough stem cell donors to meet demands of people requiring a pancreas or donated islet (insulin producing) cells. The same risks are the reason why a pancreas transplant is not carried out in people with type 1 diabetes.

Research now needs to look at ways of protecting new insulin making cells from further destruction. This could be done by a process called encapsulation, which basically means the cells are protected by a special gel like material. The protective coating has tiny microscopic holes that can let nutrients though and enable the cell to work, yet the holes are too small to let immune cells in that can attack. Think of it like a tea bag that can let the good stuff in and keep the bad stuff out.

JDRF are funding several research projects that are testing potential different materials that would form the protective coating. Generally, how the cells are protected falls into 3 categories:
- Micro encapsulation -cells are coated in a substance as described above and are only small enough to be seen under a microscope
- Macro encapsulation – insulin making cells are held in a device that is implanted into the abdomen
- Nano encapsulation – different molecules are attached to different cells; very finely coated cells are protected from the immune system yet drugs can be implanted into the cells and enhance their performance.

Regeneration of cells

Of course, cells will not need to be protected if they are not transplanted. Scientists are looking into if there is a way to get people to start growing their own beta cells again. Many events throughout the life cycle involve the production of more beta cells, such as women making more during pregnancy, or requiring more as we grow into adults. If people can make extra beta cells in these circumstances, maybe scientists can study the process and see if it is possible to encourage them to grow in the bodies of people with Type One.

Alpha cells – these grow in the pancreas alongside the beta cells, yet they remain undamaged in people with type 1. Alpha cells produce glucagon, but scientists are trying to develop a way to reprogram them to become beta cells and start making insulin. Alpha cells develop and act in the same way as beta cells, so scientists
believe it is entirely possible that one day they can be reprogrammed.

Beta Cells – it is thought that people with Type 1 still have some functioning beta cells, science could find a way to use these to regenerate the damaged beta cells.

Cells regeneration still has a long way to go before the method can be even considered as a possible cure, but the promise of further research is looking promising.

Preventing Type 1 Diabetes

JDRF understands that preventing diabetes in the first place is a great step towards their dream of a world where Type One Diabetes does not exist. In addition, if scientists can learn how to prevent it, this could give clues into why it happens and then any future research can focus on reversing it.

TrialNet

Dr Yuk-Fun Liu, University of Bristol

TrialNet is a worldwide project which analyses blood samples taken from close relatives of those with Type 1. In the UK, TrialNet is led by Dr Yuk-Fun Liu at the University of Bristol. Close relatives of people who live with Type 1 are thought to be at greater risk of developing Type 1 Diabetes themselves. TrialNet analyses the blood samples and can identify individuals that are very likely to develop Type 1, the individual is then invited to take part in a clinical trial of immunosuppressant drugs that are believed to delay or prevent Type 1. TrialNet scientists are also interested in trying to find out whether there any triggers that can contribute to the development of Type 1, by identifying these triggers we will be better informed of how to prevent it in the first place. It would then be possible to focusing research on reversing the triggers. Information gained on this study could lead researchers towards developing better treatments, or biological cures.

Early symptoms study

Dr Eoin McKinney, University of Cambridge

It is already understood that there are often signs of Type 1 Diabetes well before the symptoms develop and the immune system damages the pancreas. Dr McKinney and his team are using blood samples taken from the TrialNet study and will look at the genetic activity and try to identify any patterns that would allow doctors to easier identify who is likely to develop type 1. It is hoped that by knowing this, development of the condition could be prevented or delayed and the results could inform studies into treatments and cures.

Immune system

Dr Michael Christie, University of Lincoln

Dr Christie has teamed up with the University of Exeter to look at the role that the B cells in the immune system might play in inflammation of the pancreas, which is thought to happen just before symptoms of type 1 develop. Dr Christie wants to find out whether the B cell invasion of the pancreas accelerates the autoimmune attack, finding this out can then inform research into preventing the immune system attack that we know causes Type 1 Diabetes.

Type One Discovery Days

JDRF also host "Discovery Days" which are a great opportunity to meet other people living with Type 1 and learn more about the current research developments. Discovery Days are for all the family, children can meet others with T1 and have fun, whilst adults can listen to the talks, network and meet other parents of a child with T1.

Discovery days take place all over the UK and also in other countries, but are currently online. Discovery Days are a good opportunity to get involved with the Type 1 community in your area and find out about any events that may be on, such as fun runs, sponsored sky dives or coffee mornings! JDRF need volunteers for their events too, so you can still get involved if you do not want to run yourself.

Details of online discovery days can be found on the JDRF website.

More information about JDRF can be found online at: www.jdrf.org.uk

Chapter 12

"In 2020, no life should be at risk because they can not afford insulin"

The Pendsey Trust

It was sitting in a room in Brussels, at the European Development Days, that young journalist Lucy Laycock first heard that thousands of children internationally were dying for a lack of affordable insulin. Horrified by what she heard, particularly as her own five-year-old cousin had recently been diagnosed with the condition, she researched the topic obsessively. She was inspired to read about one man in India and his family, who had dedicated his life's work to supporting such children. His name was Dr Sharad Pendsey, and his clinic was based in Nagpur, known across India as the 'city of oranges'.

Just months later, she was on a plane to Nagpur to find out more, with funding under her belt to produce a radio documentary about this untold story. She was fascinated to learn how Dr Pendsey and his wife were inspired to establish **DREAM** Trust in 1995, after he witnessed the death of two young girls whose parents had withdrawn insulin from their children for financial reasons. Many families in Nagpur earn "daily wages" often hard labour and long working days. Already living in poverty, daily wages do not stretch to affording insulin.

Unfortunately, these were not the only tragic tales Dr Pendsey and his wife had witnessed. Lucy was shocked to hear that the cost of insulin could be as much as a third of a family's monthly income, a situation compounded by stigma and distrust of what is perceived aas "western medicine". On that visit, she met children who were banned from eating from the same plates as others, or called 'devil children' by classmates who saw them injecting themselves. The situation for women was particularly horrifying, with their value deemed worthless due to the condition. Unfortunately, they are perceived as poor marriage partners, and thus become a burden to their families. Consequences of a lack of regular insulin and medical care were also apparent, with children displaying stunted growth, abscesses, and reporting regular hospitalisation for diabetic ketoacidosis.

Dr Pendsey's work is nothing short of inspirational. An internationally esteemed endocrinologist, alongside his private work he provides free medical care for Type 1 diabetes patients at the clinic. No patient is turned away, irrespective of their ability to pay. This includes a full package, not only of insulin provision but counselling and education about the importance of careful management of the condition. In addition, and perhaps most significantly, the clinic aims to enable the patients to live with pride and dignity, fighting stigma still faced in society. This includes scholarships for schooling and vocational courses, to enable the young people to one day become self-sufficient for their medical costs. The clinic even helps women to secure successful marriages by educating their partners, and numerous patients have become the envy of their communities by entering prestigious professions such as nursing under Dr Pendsey's guidance.

Lucy was struck by the poverty she witnessed, and the plight of one particular young girl imprinted on her mind. Then only eight years old, the newly diagnosed girl lived in a very basic home, constructed of wattle and mud. Her father was unable to work due to health issues, and her mother was struggling to provide for her family as a daily labourer in the countryside. The family lived many miles from the clinic in a rural village with little infrastructure. How could such a family overcome her diagnosis?

On returning to the UK, Lucy was determined to help Dr Pendsey and his patients to achieve their dreams. With a few friends, she started holding fundraising events in London, and soon was able to establish a UK registered charity (no 1158007) inspired by his work - The Pendsey Trust. The focus of the charity is twofold - to support the provision of insulin and medical supplies to the those who need it most, but equally to enable Dr Pendsey's vocational and educational programme to develop and provide a more sustainable future for those at the clinic. This two pronged approach is effective as it addresses the immediate need whilst also solving the long term problems of poverty and gender inequality.

The charity has continued to grow and flourish, largely through word of mouth and social media. The Pendsey Trust currently support over 100 children full time through the child sponsorship programme, with families in the UK enjoying the experience of linking with families in India. Many of our families in the UK consider their sponsor child as a member of their family, some have even visited India (at their own expense) to meet their child and many other children who are helped by the trust.

Countless young people have also been supported to attend school and even university, alongside provision of travel grants where needed. Many patients have been able to access vocational tools, training, and business start-ups, from sewing machines to start a tailoring business, food carts to start a street food business to buffalo farming!

The charity has also supported numerous initiatives created by DREAM Trust, such as the bicycle project. The first bicycle project involved shipping 100 recycled bicycles from the UK to Nagpur. The bicycles were donated, repaired and shipped to India to enable individuals to reach school or the clinic from remote areas. Many of the Pendsey Trust's children live in remote villages and travelling to school can be many miles away over rough terrain. In 45c heat and with diabetes thrown into the mix, this can make it very hard for the child to get to school. A simple bicycle overcomes this problem.

Perhaps most uniquely, the charity continues to be run entirely by volunteers, most with a link to T1D, with Lucy remaining determined that every single penny raised should be transferred to India and not be spent on administration.

Lucy continues to return to India on a self-funded basis once every few years, most recently celebrating her wedding in Indian style with clinic staff. Like many of the sponsor families in the UK, she considers the staff and patients to be her extended family, being inspired by their bravery and determination.

Amazing developments over the years have transformed the clinic's operation, with Dr Pendsey's ability to adapt rapidly to maximise the standard of care received by the patients. An enormous improvement has been the introduction of electricity to many of the poor areas in which the children live, this has enabled The Pendsey Trust to provide funding for fridges for families to store insulin safely in India's long hot summers. All children were also provided with a Frio bag, this keeps insulin cool either throughout the day, or all the time if the child still lives in a village with no electricity.

Most recently, The Pendsey Trust has been fundraising to support the clinic as patients face worrying economic times during the Covid-19 epidemic.

Amazingly, Lucy and her family were able to sponsor the medical care of the small girl she met on her first visit, who is now a very talkative and determined 17-year-old girl, hoping to pursue a career in nursing. This amazing young lady is now one of hundreds of The Pendsey Trust's success stories.

The Pendsey Trust's partner clinic are proud to announce the following:

- 2000 children are now provided with insulin at the clinic

- Mostly, the children are provided with human insulin, although 20-30% still take a short and long acting analogue insulin

- All children are provided with a blood glucose meter to test with, as well as strips and lancets. Most children can now test 8 – 10 times a week.

- Over 950 bicycles have been provided to children to enable them to travel to school safely, without this help it can be difficult for the children to access school as it can be far away and involve difficult terrain

- Refridgeration can also be a problem, over 256 fridges have been provided to date and 400 Frio bags

- Educational scholarships are provided to around 500 children annually. Scholarship amounts can range from 10,000 to 20,000 Indian Rupees, which is approx. £100 to £200, or US$133 - $266.

- Business start up grants and support are provided for approximately 30 young people per year, the value is 15,000 – 25,000 Indian Rupees, or £150 to £250, or US$200 to $335 each.

- Children are also provided with a school bag, over 500 of these are provided annually as such a small thing can really make a difference in the life of a child going to school.

Currently, The Pendsey Trust are appealing for help to provide families with emergency Covid grants. Life is difficult for those with Type 1 diabetes in the developing world in normal times, but strict lockdowns and mass business closures caused by Covid-19 have thrown many families into economic ruin. Many of these families were already struggling and living on the breadline, despite being very hard workers.

Whilst the Indian government is providing emergency rations, most of the families Pendsey Trust work with live below the poverty line and take daily wages, which is no longer viable in the current situation. Insulin costs as much as half of a poor family's monthly income in a normal situation, and now families are battling a complete loss of income, the permanent destruction of their small businesses, and difficulties accessing their usual sources of medication.

The Pendsey trust are proud to be run entirely by volunteers who donate their time and skills to enable every penny that is donated to reach the children in India. This means they have a "no admin" policy and every penny donated can be accounted for and will only fund sustainable initiatives that enhance the live of a person living with Type 1. Every penny can also be accounted for in India too, as patients are fully vetted and referenced to ensure those in the most need of help receive it. Communication between India and England is excellent, making sure everyone is accountable. Learn more about how we can account for every penny in our blog post "Every Penny Counts" which can be found here:
http://www.thependseytrust.org/every-penny-counts/

A little goes a long way in India:

£4 buys one week of insulin
£5 can provide a travel grant to clinic
£10 buys a school uniform, school bag and bag to keep insulin in for a child to attend school
£12 buys a Frio bag and this could be the only way a person can keep their insulin cool
£16 provides life saving insulin for a month
£40 can pay for school for a year
£40 buys a bicycle for a child to safely get to school
£50 provides emergency medical supplies due to covid

£80 can buy a sewing machine to enable a young person to start a tailoring business

£100 can fund a young person to attend college

£150 can allow a young person to start a business, making them independent with insulin costs

Please check the website at **www.thependseytrust.org** or the Facebook page at **www.facebook.com/thependseytrust** for further information about the trust, how you can help and to keep up to date with current and future campaigns.

The Pendsey Trust would also be very grateful for likes and shares on their social media, this helps us keep to our costs down by not paying for ad's or to boost posts, thus helping us stick to our "no admin" policy.

Glossary

Basal - basal refers to long acting insulin that usually works over 24 hours. Basal insulin is also known as "background" insulin and it ensures the body always has some insulin. Basal is injected once or twice a day and examples of basal insulin are Tresiba, Lantus and Levimir. If a person uses a pump, instead of injecting the pump constantly drips insulin, acting as bolus.

Bolus - bolus refers to faster acting insulin that is usually given at meal times or to treat high blood sugars. Bolus examples are Fiasp and Novorapid. If a person uses a pump, they can bolus via the pump, giving it an instruction of how much insulin to deliver with the meal or to correct a high.

Blood Glucose or BG - this is the amount of sugar in the blood

Continuous Glucose Monitor or CGM - this is a device worn by a person with diabetes to continually measure their blood glucose, the information is bluetoothed to a handset, phone or even insulin pump. A CGM takes away the need to finger prick so can mean increased testing and better control. Some devices can alarm when a hypo is near.

Dexcom - a trade name of the CGM

DKA or Diabetic Keto Acidosis - this is a serious medical problem that starts developing when the body runs out of insulin. It leads to coma and can be fatal.

Flash Glucose Monitor or FGM - similar to CGM, except an FGM measures the blood when a device or phone (with a special app) is waved over it. An FGM can take away the need to finger prick and lead to better control.

Gluco-meter - a hand held machine that can measure how much sugar is in the blood

HBa1c - this is a special type of blood test usually performed in clinic and is a great indicator of the overall control of diabetes. Many people with Type 1 Diabetes see it as their "report card".

Hypoglycaemia or "hypo" - this happens when there is not enough sugar in the blood (below 4) and is a medical emergency that needs treating with fast acting sugar. Symptoms of hypo include dizziness, paleness, shaking, seizures, sweating and behavioural problems.

Hyperglycaemia or "hyper" - high blood sugars, if above 14mmol this can lead to DKA, in addition, the compound effect of regular elevated blood sugars can also damage vision, heart, kidneys and cause problems with the feet resulting in amputation, blindness and organ failure. Symtpoms of hyperglycaemia include frequent urination, excessive thirst, weight loss, hunger, dry skin and fatigue. Hyperglycaemia can only be treated with insulin.

Ketones - these are chemicals in the blood caused by lack of insulin and the body burning its own fat, this is highly dangerous for people with diabetes and it is the first sign the body is going into DKA. Thankfully, a different type of blood test is available that the person can do to see if they have ketones developing and if they do, can treat with extra insulin and/or medical advice.

Libre - a flash glucose monitor made by Abbott Diabetes

Multiple Daily Injections (MDI) - this refers to the multiple daily injections a person living with diabetes has to do. People who chose to manage their condition via an insulin pump do not have to do MDI but they still have to learn how to do it in case the pump fails and would still be expected to do MDI in some emergency situations.

Omnipod - a tubeless insulin pump

PDM or Personal Diabetes Manager - this is the handset that comes with an Omnipod, the user gives the PDM instructions so the Omnipod knows what to do and when

Acknowledgements

Huge thanks to all the awesome people who agreed to take part in this book and tell their story. I understand that telling your stories can sometimes be emotional, but I really appreciate your input. I am certain that telling your stories has helped other parents to feel reassured. This book is also to highlight you as individuals, share your successes and acknowledge the hurdles you have had to leap over to get there. Well done!

I would like to thank all the fellow T1 Parents who "just get it." Many of you have supported me over the years, providing advice, friendship and solidarity at all times of the day and night. Thanks also for your support with this book.

I am overwhelmed by the support of everyone who has helped and offered support during the writing of this publication. Once again, this is a testament to the Type 1 Community; a club we didn't chose to be part of, one we would never want to join, but now we are in it we are not on our own as we are supported by some amazing people.

Special thanks go to:
Auntie Mary, Debbie, Karen, Jo, Reba, and anyone else I forgot for their help with proof-reading, editing, formatting and drafting out this book.

Massive thanks to Linda for the design of the book cover, who has been amazing and very supportive throughout. If you are looking for any graphics then please get in touch with her at
https://www.facebook.com/wearevisualimpact

We highly recommend ARC for remote office and virtual PA services and thank them for their assistance with this book.
arcvirtualpaservices.com

Printed in Great Britain
by Amazon